THE COMPLETE IDIOT'S GUIDE® TO

Body Ball Fitness

Illustrated

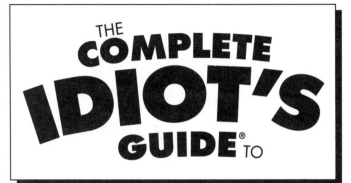

Body Ball Fitness

Illustrated

by Karon Karter

ALPHA

A member of Penguin Group (USA) Inc.

To my family

ALPHA BOOKS

Published by the Penguin Group

Penguin Group (USA) Inc., 375 Hudson Street, New York, New York 10014, U.S.A.

Penguin Group (Canada), 10 Alcorn Avenue, Toronto, Ontario, Canada M4V 3B2 (a division of Pearson Penguin Canada Inc.)

Penguin Books Ltd, 80 Strand, London WC2R 0RL, England

Penguin Ireland, 25 St Stephen's Green, Dublin 2, Ireland (a division of Penguin Books Ltd)

Penguin Group (Australia), 250 Camberwell Road, Camberwell, Victoria 3124, Australia (a division of Pearson Australia Group Pty Ltd)

Penguin Books India Pvt Ltd, 11 Community Centre, Panchsheel Park, New Delhi—110 017, India

Penguin Group (NZ), Cnr Airborne and Rosedale Roads, Albany, Auckland, New Zealand (a division of Pearson New Zealand Ltd)

Penguin Books (South Africa) (Pty) Ltd, 24 Sturdee Avenue, Rosebank, Johannesburg 2196, South Africa

Penguin Books Ltd, Registered Offices: 80 Strand, London WC2R 0RL, England

Copyright © 2004 by Karon Karter

International Standard Book Number: 1-59257-266-9
Library of Congress Catalog Card Number: 2004110009

06   05   04   8   7   6   5   4   3   2   1

Interpretation of the printing code: The rightmost number of the first series of numbers is the year of the book's printing; the rightmost number of the second series of numbers is the number of the book's printing. For example, a printing code of 04-1 shows that the first printing occurred in 2004.

Printed in the United States of America

Note: This publication contains the opinions and ideas of its author. It is intended to provide helpful and informative material on the subject matter covered. It is sold with the understanding that the author and publisher are not engaged in rendering professional services in the book. If the reader requires personal assistance or advice, a competent professional should be consulted.

The author and publisher specifically disclaim any responsibility for any liability, loss, or risk, personal or otherwise, which is incurred as a consequence, directly or indirectly, of the use and application of any of the contents of this book.

Most Alpha books are available at special quantity discounts for bulk purchases for sales promotions, premiums, fund-raising, or educational use. Special books, or book excerpts, can also be created to fit specific needs.

For details, write: Special Markets, Alpha Books, 375 Hudson Street, New York, NY 10014.

Publisher: *Marie Butler-Knight*
Product Manager: *Phil Kitchel*
Senior Managing Editor: *Jennifer Chisholm*
Senior Acquisitions Editor: *Randy Ladenheim-Gil*
Senior Development Editor: *Tom Stevens*
Senior Production Editor: *Billy Fields*
Copy Editor: *Jennifer Connolly*
Illustrator: *Richard King*
Cover/Book Designer: *Trina Wurst*
Indexer: *Julie Bess*
Layout: *Becky Harmon*
Proofreading: *Mary Hunt*

Contents at a Glance

Part 1: Body and the Ball 2

   1   Ballercise 4

Why and how the ball will benefit you, plus guidelines on how to size your ball along with precautions.

   2   A Balanced Ball Body 10

To help you get ready for your ball workouts, here's a look at what fitness is and how you can get fit using the ball.

   3   Body Ball Wisdom 18

You will learn all about posture and why it's vital to your good health and good looks, plus a look at your anatomy in-depth so you can be ready for the ball workouts.

Part 2: Get Your Best Ball Body 26

   4   Beginner Ball Bliss 28

Holding yourself high on the ball begins by strengthening the muscles that support your spine. Because the ball is dynamic, this beginner workout develops postural strength and stability. You'll first instinctively train your body, and then develop plenty of strength to stay on the ball.

   5   The Body Ball Makeover 46

As your postural muscles keep you afloat, you'll move your arms and legs to challenge your stability on the ball even more in this intermediate workout.

   6   Mind-Body Ball Blitz 68

This workout is a collection of exercises that are meant to challenge your balance and strength at the same time. These exercises require using multiple muscles and lots of balance so you can move toward your best ball body.

Part 3: It's a Mind-Body Ball Thing 86

   7   The Poised Pilates Ball Body 88

This chapter shows you a whole new way to workout on the ball and why the ball and Pilates work well together.

   8   Mind-Bending Ball Workout 96

You can experience a Pilates on the ball workout in this chapter, using some of the traditional exercises designed by Joseph Pilates.

Part 4: **Restorative Ball** 118

   9   Body Ball Therapy 120

Got an aching back? Then read about how you may reduce the back blues, plus you can try to do a gentle ball back workout, which was designed by physical therapist, Karen Sanzo.

  10 Stressed? Then Stretch Over the Ball! 138

Stressed Out? Here's your chance to relax, renew, and restore your body with ball stretches.

Appendixes

   A   Glossary 158

   B   Quick Workouts: Multi-Muscle Training 163

   C   Quick Workouts: Abdominal Training..167

   D   Beat Belly Fat with the Ball 171

   E   Myths and Mysteries about Abdominal Training 175

       Index 177

Contents

Part 1: Body and the Ball 2

  1 Ballercise 4

      Functional Fitness 5

      Overcoming the Plateau State 7

      The Right Ball for You 8

      Test-driving Your Ball 8

      On the Ball Precautions 8

  2 A Balanced Ball Body 10

      A Balanced Body 11

        Cardiorespiratory Fitness 12

        Strength 12

        Flexibility 13

      The Fat Factor 13

      Ball Fitness 13

      The Ball and Beyond 14

        Balance Training 14

        Postural Training 14

        Body Sense Training 15

      On or Off the Ball 16

  3 Body Ball Wisdom 18

      Posture Performance (the Truth) 19

      Back Basics 20

      Navigating Neutral 20

      Pelvis Perfection 21

      Shoulder Smarts 22

      Middle Muscles That Matter 23

      Hippity-Hop or Hippity-Flop? 24

      Before You Begin 25

Part 2: Get Your Best Ball Body 26

  4 Beginner Ball Bliss 28

      Ball Basics: Beginner Exercises 29

      Seated Ball Postural Exercises: Finding a Neutral Spine on the Ball 30

      Seated Ball Postural Exercises: Ball Rocking 32

      Seated Ball Postural Exercises: Leg and Arm Raises 34

      Squat off the Ball 36

Walking down the Ball 37
Abdominal Ball Curls 38
Supine Ball Bridge 39
Spinal Ball Extension 40
Drape over the Ball 41
Cross Ball Extension 42
Stationary Ball Plank 43
Ball Bridge on the Floor 44
Congratulations! 45

5   The Body Ball Makeover 46
The Total Body Ball Makeover: Ball Intermediates 47
Seated Ball Biceps Curl 49
Seated Ball Triceps Extension 50
Seated Ball Front Raise 51
Seated Ball Lateral Raise 52
Seated Ball Bent-Over Fly 53
Supine Ball Bridge with Chest Press 54
Supine Ball Bridge with Fly 55
Spinal Ball Extension 56
Spinal Ball Extension with Leg Lift 57
One Arm Standing Row with Ball 58
Abdominal Ball Curl 59
Abdominal Ball Oblique Curl 60
Stationary Ball Plank 61
Ball Wall Squat 62
Ball Pliè Wall Squat 64
Ball Sideline Outer Thigh Work 65
Ball Bridge with Leg Curl 66
Congratulations 67

6   Mind-Body Ball Blitz 68
Mind–Body Ball Blitz: Advanced 69
Ball Wall Squat with Biceps Curl 71
Ball Pliè Wall Squat with Upright Row 72
Ball Single Leg Lunge 73
One Arm Standing Row with Single Leg Ball Squat 74
Stationary Ball Plank 75
Stationary Ball Plank with Leg Extension 76
Stationary Ball Pike 77
Stationary Ball Push-Up 78
Spinal Ball Extension 79
Spinal Ball Extension with Triceps Kickback 80

Ball Bridge with Leg Curls and Leg Extensions 81
Inner Thigh Ball Squeeze with Abdominal Curl 83
Reverse Ball Curl 84
Scissor Ball Rotation 85

Part 3:   It's a Mind–Body Ball Thing **86**

7   The Poised Pilates Ball Body 88
Defining Pilates? 89
The Beginning: Joseph Pilates 90
The Awesome Twosome! 90
The Heart of Pilates 91
Concentration *92*
Control *92*
Centering *92*
Flow *92*
Precision *92*
Breathing *93*
Lateral Breathing Exercises 94
Pilates on the Ball 95

8   Mind-Bending Ball Workout 96
The Pilates Plan 97
The Fab Five 98
The Pilates "V" 98
The Hundred 99
The Rollup 101
Leg Circles 103
Rolling Like a Ball 105
Single-Leg Stretch 107
Double-Leg Stretch 109
Spine Stretch 110
The Saw 111
Side Kick Ball Series: Kick Front and Back, Leg Ball Circles,
    and Ball Beats 113
Side Kick Ball Series: Leg Ball Circles 114
Side Kick Ball Series: Ball Beats 115
Seal 117

Part 4:   Restorative Ball **118**

9   Body Ball Therapy 120
Back in Business 121
Identifying the Trained Eye 122

Lumbar Low Down 123
Back Matters 123
Fighting Back the Back Blues 124
Don't Get On the Ball 124
The Fifteen-Minute Back Solution 125
Lower Back Stretch (Subtle Pelvic Tilts) 126
Moving Legs with Stable Spine (Feet on Ball) 127
Hamstring Stretch 128
Pectoral and Latissimus Stretch 129
Seated Spine Stretch 130
Seated Pelvic Tilts 131
Seated Hip Flexion to Seated Knee Extension 132
Small Rotation with Neutral Spine 133
Plank (Added Challenge) 135
Raise Ball Overhead 136
Lasting Therapy 137

10   Stressed? Then Stretch Over the Ball! 138
Renew, Relax, and Restore 139
Restorative Ball 140
The Restorative Plan 140
Seated Neck Stretch 141
Seated Back Stretch 142
Seated Chest Stretch...142
Pectoral Stretch 143
Seated Rotation Stretch 144
Seated Lateral Trunk Stretch 145
Supine Arm Circles 146
Hamstrings Stretch 147
Spinal Twist 148
Adductor Stretch 149
Lower Back Stretch 149
Gluteal Stretch 150
Thread the Needle Stretch 150
Sideline Stretch 151
Prone Quadriceps Stretch 152
Supine Spinal Traction 153
Seated Buttocks and Hamstrings Stretch 154
Standing Back Stretch 155
Standing Shoulder Stretch at Wall 155
Seated Neck Stretch 156
Supine Spinal Traction 156

Appendixes

A Glossary 158

B Quick Workouts: Multi-Muscle Training 163

C Quick Workouts: Just Abs! 167

D Beat Belly Fat with the Ball 171

E Myths and Mysteries About Abdominal Training 175

   Index 177

Foreword

As a group exercise instructor, personal trainer, and group exercise coordinator for the Baylor Tom Landry Fitness Center, I have been working in the fitness profession for more than 20 years. About five years ago, I attended a convention for fitness professionals and went to a workshop presented by Stephanie and Mike Morris. They had developed a program using Resist-a-Balls, big round balls that looked like something I played with as a child. I walked in the room and everyone was trying different exercises on the ball. I was not sure what I was walking into. The dilemma was that when I tried the exercises, I could not do them. I have competed in bodybuilding and competitive aerobics and I was strong—there was not much that I couldn't do—but I could not seem to find the balance and strength necessary to perform the exercises that Stephanie and Mike were demonstrating.

Then I heard the phrase "core strength," and I soon realized that I was strong in my extremities, upper body, and legs but was missing the all-important core strength—the strength that comes from the abdominals, lower back and shoulder area. From that point on I was determined to develop my core strength. I did the exercises and practiced them faithfully and slowly but surely was able to master the exercises. Along the way, I noticed I didn't have recurring pain in my low back as I did before when I lifted weights. I was standing a little taller with better posture; I seemed as strong on one leg as I was on two; and I could add weights and still get on the ball and challenge myself.

In the end, I have a stronger and more functional body that enables me do the activities I want and helps me prevent injuries.

This book will help *you* develop *your* core strength. The book takes you through the beginning moves and adds challenges to your body as you develop more strength. Karon's knowledge of the body and her ability to detail the exercises in a way that everyone can understand will help you gain your own core strength. This book should be an important part of everyone's fitness program.

So what are you waiting for? Get on the ball!

—Marilyn Levitt, group exercise coordinator at the Baylor Tom Landry Fitness Center.

Introduction

You look good, yet sense that you could look even better: How can I get the most out of my workout? How can I reach my body's full potential?

So you're itching for a little workout inspiration—new challenges to shape up your body and soul. That's where body ball fitness comes in. Fitness ball is the latest craze to roll out! You can develop amazing muscles from head to toe, enhance your body like no other fitness, and stretch your mind for the journey of a lifetime. It's a balancing act worth trying especially if you're longing for a new you.

In this book, you have a variety of ball exercises to pick from. If you're longing to get stronger or lose those last few inches, these workouts will transform your current workout into a result-driven workout.

Fitness Ball is an effective, inexpensive, and versatile piece of equipment. Whether you're a regular gym-goer, elite athlete, or first timer, Body Ball can be easily adapted to meet your needs. You can increase or decrease the intensity of a movement depending on your physical training, age, or how comfortable you are exercising on a ball. You can use dumbbell weights on the ball to increase the intensity or enjoy a restorative stretch on the ball—it's up to you!

How This Book Is Organized

Whether you want to tweak your torso or fine-tune your body, the pages in this book roll several workouts into one: You can enjoy a complete muscle makeover or a soothing stretch. This book offers a little something for everyone. Here's a quick overview:

Part 1, "Body and the Ball," introduces you to the ball. As you read on, you will find out why it's so important and how you can get more from it. These chapters get you ready for your body ball workouts.

Part 2, "Get Your Best Ball Body," offers you three total body ball workouts varying in degrees of difficulty to keep you and your muscles challenged for some time. Each workout was designed to give you a total body makeover so you can move toward your best ball body—strong and sculpted.

Part 3, "It's a Mind Body Ball Thing," introduces you to Pilates on the ball! In this part, you learn a little about Pilates, why the ball and Pilates make an awesome twosome, and then transform poochy abs into amazing ones with a Pilates on the ball workout.

Part 4, "Restorative Ball," gives you an opportunity to relax, renew, and restore your body with ball exercises that offer both back and body relief.

Extras

This book has a number of informative sidebars that provide additional tips on exercising, the ball, definitions, and precautions.

On the Ball

Check out these sidebars for common tips, hints, and other valuable information. This sidebar enhances your ball journey.

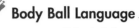

Body Ball Language

Here you'll find definitions of terms used in this book so that you can use them on the ball or in the gym and expand your exercise knowledge.

Ball Blowout

These precautions warn you of common mishaps on the ball.

Acknowledgments

I'm so grateful to my acquisitions editor, Randy Landenheim-Gil. Thank you for trusting me enough to hire me over and over again. Of course, there is the entire team from Alpha Books that I must thank including my development editor, Tom Stevens and Billy Fields, senior production editor. Thank you both for painstakingly and patiently sorting through many, many exercise steps and photos to make this book perfect—and, of course, Jennifer Connolly, my copy editor, for fine tuning my words to perfection. I'm grateful to the entire team of Alpha—you guys are the best!

At home, I'm completely indebted to many people. First, thank you, Karen Sanzo so much for being part of this project and taking time off from your busy schedule to provide technical and emotional support during the photo shoot. I've learned so much from you over the years—you are my inspirational vehicle to keep learning and growing as a person and instructor! Thank you, Paul Schoenberg, General Manager of Premier Athletic Club, for opening your doors so that I could shoot my pictures. And then there is Beth Smith from the Baylor Tom Landry Shop for providing such wonderful clothing. I'm completely grateful to Danny Turning. You are such a gifted photographer, and I'm so happy that we had the opportunity to work together many years ago, because here we are today. Thanks to you and your assistant for your time and patience during the shoot and the editing process, which seemed endless. Suzi Grey—four books later and you're still doing my makeup and hair! I'm so fortunate that we met many, many years ago because I can always count on you to transform my face for the oh-so-better.

As always, I owe a ton of gratitude to my writing coach, Janet Harris. Even though she insists that I don't need her any longer, I won't write without her! And then there's Kubera, my adorable Tibetan Spaniel. He keeps me company day after day while I write behind closed doors and is a women's best friend. Thank you, Kjehl Rasmussen, for keeping my best interest at heart. Of course, there wouldn't be any books if I didn't have the support from my family.

Trademarks

All terms mentioned in this book that are known to be or are suspected of being trademarks or service marks have been appropriately capitalized. Alpha Books and Penguin Group (USA) Inc. cannot attest to the accuracy of this information. Use of a term in this book should not be regarded as affecting the validity of any trademark or service mark.

In This Part

1 Ballercise

2 The Balanced Ball Body

3 Body Ball Wisdom

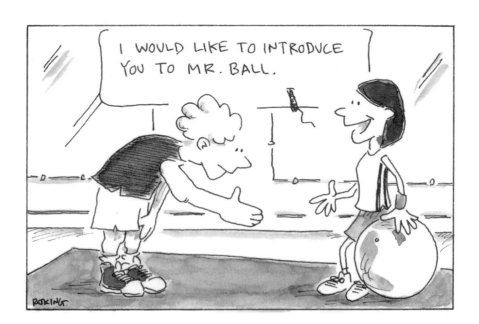

Part 1

Body and the Ball

In this part, I introduce you to the ball, its importance, and how to get more of it. The ball is a balancing act worth trying whether you're looking for a way to reinvigorate your workouts or a whole new way to workout. This book offers something for everyone. You can try the ball workouts, which cover a full range of ball exercises to strengthen, stretch, and sculpt your body.

In This Chapter

- ◆ Why the ball?
- ◆ Benefits of the ball
- ◆ Sizing your ball
- ◆ Ball precautions

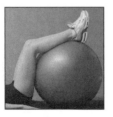 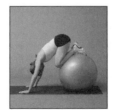 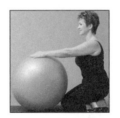 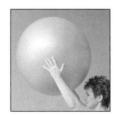 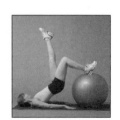

Chapter 1

Ballercise

Let's face it: You can't wish yourself thin! But you can get off the couch and on the ball for workouts that offer ultra-amazing body results. Even if you love counting the caloric burn, adding up the reps, and watching the "LBs" melt (and who wouldn't), your workout might scream semi-automatic. So, wouldn't you love to rev up the body results? That's where this book comes in. Sure, body ball fitness tells you how to use the latest trend in exercise, but this book will also pump up any old rep session and center your workout, striking the perfect balance between abs of steel and a body of head-to-toe steel.

Functional Fitness

Even though the fitness ball is up-to-the-minute fresh, it has been around for about 40 years. The first recorded use of the ball was treating patients with spinal injuries in Switzerland during the 1960s. About 10 years ago, the fitness industry caught sight of the ball and soon found that its versatility made it available piece of exercise equipment. And today physical therapists use the ball to treat back injuries.

In any given workout you must use multiple muscle groups to incorporate stability and balance challenges, and the ball is used to coordinate the body's entire musculature to achieve more balance and strength. Of course, working out on the ball has so many other benefits, the least of which is an amazing body, but the body ball delivers an even bigger result: It strengthens your body to meet your daily demands. Enter *functional fitness!*

Functional fitness builds strength in movement, training the body to be spatially aware of its position at any given moment. Today's trend is strengthening your body so that it meets your real life activities. Functional fitness is a term now endorsed by the American Council of Exercise (ACE), which is the largest fitness certifying body for personal trainers and fitness instructors.

Performance isn't reserved for the gym. Life is your performance and it alternates between bouts of cardio and bouts of strength: The ability to balance your baby on your left knee while trying to eat with your right hand; the skills to spike a volleyball and then land on both feet; the sprint-like power to jump between two near-closing doors of your commuter train; and the strength to shovel the heavy wet-like snow after a major blizzard are examples of real life movements occurring every day. Some movements are repetitive while others are full-blown power moves. Wouldn't it be nice to have enough strength to perform them all safely?

Gym machines are fine, but a problem arises with strengthening your muscles on traditional weight machines; they are often one-size-fits-all, working only one muscle at a time and in isolation. Moreover, most traditional weight machines were built for bodybuilders. However, if body building is your goal, then you're training as you should be. If, however, you just want enough strength to make it through your day safely along with great body tone, you don't have to train like a bodybuilder to get functional strength.

Because the ball is wobbly, you engage multiple muscles to keep it steady underneath you. This integrated approach to physical training is more in line with your day-to-day activities. A functional exercise on the ball, for example, can challenge your abdominal and back muscles to maintain your center of gravity on the ball in just about every exercise. Eventually, this strength carries over to your every day life.

As a result, ball exercises are more challenging at least at first. After all, sitting on a moving surface is harder than sitting in a stationary chair. Yet it's worth the ride, especially if you're adding up the calories used to activate all of those muscles in any given exercise. In other words, you can inspire a lot of muscles in these ball workouts so visible fat melts away.

On the Ball

Fitness ball develops your strength through stability and balance challenges while integrating several muscle groups at the same time.

In addition, you quickly learn to sit with good posture, engaging your middle muscles including your abdominals and back muscles because they keep you afloat. There are many benefits of the fitness ball worth looking at:

- Strengthens your body as a whole, incorporating an integrated approach to fitness
- Engages your core muscles, while strengthening your arms and legs simultaneously in just about every exercise
- Improves posture through the development of a certain amount of body awareness
- Builds balancing skills because the body and brain work together to keep the ball steady underneath
- Shrinks inches from your body
- Burns calories because you're asking your muscles to do more in any given exercise
- Offers a greater range of motion so you can do exercises in a variety of positions
- Improves your body sense and coordination because of the wobbly nature of the ball
- Improves flexibility and joint mobility because it can be used as a prop to increase a stretch

- Adapts workouts to individual physical needs—modify or intensify an exercise by shortening or lengthening your limbs away from the ball, which acts as a fulcrum
- Becomes your most versatile piece of exercise equipment because the ball lifts you off the floor so you can exercise or stretch in a variety of positions—sitting, reclining forward, stretching backward or sideways, kneeling, and if you're a super dare devil, standing
- It's fun!

Overcoming the Plateau State

If you've seen very little change in your body—the dreaded *plateau state*—it's not because your exercise routine is completely worthless. Even the best routines get old to your body as your muscles quickly learn to bob and weave around any challenges thrown their way. Muscles get bored, so you don't see any new body results. You can, however, alter your workout ever so slightly to keep your muscles guessing, which is where the ball comes in. You can do the same exercise on the ball as you were doing in your gym, yet that same exercise becomes a new challenge for your muscles. Think about it: Your body must learn how to keep the ball from rolling out from underneath you while training multiple muscles, requiring much more muscle power, which provides your body with a whole new challenge.

Body Ball Language

Plateau state is the body's adaptation to an exercise routine, halting further muscle development or tone.

In general, there are a variety of ways to increase the intensity to prevent your body from adapting: You can add more weight, do more repetitions, or add more minutes to your gym time. But if those options don't appeal to you, the ball can work just as well to overhaul your workout.

The Right Ball for You

There are a variety of balls on the market varying in color, size, and quality. There are two kinds of balls: anti-burst balls and balls that burst. If a ball bursts while you're on top, you might injure yourself falling to the floor. Obviously, balls that burst are not as safe, but they're less expensive if that's a consideration. On the other hand, anti-burst balls are a little steadier and maintain their shape and size for many years.

> **Ball Blowout**
>
> Clean your ball from time to time, especially if you're prone to sweating or working out with lotion or oil on your body. To clean your ball, mix a little warm water and soap and then wipe it down with a soft cloth. Store your ball in any room in your house, but avoid extreme heat. You may not want your ball rolling over something printed in black ink such as a newspaper because it permanently marks your ball.

Test-driving Your Ball

As you search for the right ball, take into consideration your height. Finding the right size for you is not tricky, but your goal is to find a comfortable fit. Most people use a medium sized ball (55cm). However, depending on the manufacturing, that actual size may vary, so don't be afraid to test-drive your ball: Sit on top of it, bounce it, and stretch over it!

While sitting, make sure your knees fall even with or slightly above your hips. When bouncing on it, keep in mind that a firm ball increases the intensity of the exercise, while a softer ball lessens the intensity.

If you're de-conditioned, overweight, or mature in age, you may consider using a larger, softer ball. You can always get another ball later if you need more of a challenge. Depending on the manufacturer, balls come in three different sizes, but you should buy a ball that feels good to you:

◆ 45cm

◆ 55cm

◆ 65cm

> **On the Ball**
>
> You can inflate your ball with a bicycle pump, an electric air compressor, or the pump specifically designed for your ball. When inflating, add enough air until your ball is firm because inevitably some air will leak out while disengaging the pump.

On the Ball Precautions

Keep in mind that the fitness ball increases the intensity of any workout because it wobbles, so please use your best judgment. Regardless of whether you're a fitness buff or a first timer, ball exercises are challenging and take some time to learn. Below are a few precautions:

◆ Always consult your physician before starting any exercise program.

◆ If you have any pain while exercising, then please stop immediately.

◆ Exercise in a big area so you won't roll into a sharp object such as the edge of a coffee table.

- Invest in a good mat. If you fall off the ball—and it's a very real possibility—then it won't hurt as much with the protection of a soft mat.
- Don't exercise on a slippery surface.
- Exercise at your level of fitness. The exercises in this book are divided into beginner, intermediate, and advanced. Don't rush ahead thinking that you're more advance than you really are because you might get injured. Not training correctly or improper body alignment will only hinder your progress.
- Always warm up with a cardio workout before these workouts, such as walking, running, swimming, bicycling, or cardio machines.

Ball Blowout

All balls are not equal. Buy a burst-resistant or anti-burst ball whenever possible. The difference between the burst-balls and nonburst balls is rather obvious, but consider this: If a sharp object punctures a burst-ball, it deflates quickly, dropping you to the floor. If a burst-resistance ball is punctured, then the ball deflates slowly. Fitness balls are available at most local sporting goods stores or back rehabilitation stores.

The Least You Need to Know

- Stability ball is the latest craze; it's a balancing act worth trying, especially if you want to tweak your torso and fine-tune your upper and lower body.
- Basic ball principles, combined with strength conditioning, provide an exceptional workout that is relatively inexpensive to do.
- Because the ball is wobbly, you'll draw on extra muscles and develop new skills.
- Body balls deliver functional fitness—training your body so it is spatially aware of its position at any given moment.
- The ball comes in three different sizes: 45cm, 55cm, and 65cm.
- Ball fitness is an effective, inexpensive, and versatile workout that anyone can do, regardless of your fitness level, age, or current training.

In This Chapter

- ◆ What is fitness?
- ◆ Balanced ball body
- ◆ Balance and beyond
- ◆ Overhaul your workout with the ball

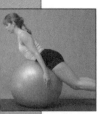
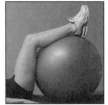
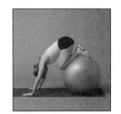
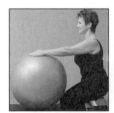
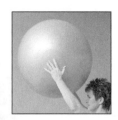
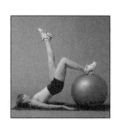

Chapter 2

A Balanced Ball Body

Getting fit hasn't always been easy. Diets *du jour* along with fad fitness methods can leave you confused rather than conditioned. Still, it seems that every fit-pro has an opinion as to what fitness is. This chapter sets the record straight and tells you how to get fit using the ball.

A Balanced Body

Must we "thigh master" our legs thin, have the stamina of a marathoner, or have the strength of a Monday night quarterback to be fit? Not exactly!

Fitness improves your overall health so that you can enjoy your life with plenty of energy, not artificial energy—like the energy you get from hourly sprints to Starbucks—but real energy that puts some spring in your step. If you're fit, you feel better, and your body has the ability to fight some of today's most debilitating diseases, such as heart disease. Best of all, if you're fit, you look great because you're moving toward a healthier you.

Can a ball keep you fit? You bet! Because the ball enhances whatever fitness routine you may be doing, you can add it to develop new skills and put a new spin on some old moves.

According to The American College of Sports Medicine (ACSM), one of the world's largest exercise certifying bodies and exercise science associations, your weekly fitness routine should include three elements—the big "3":

♦ Cardiorespiratory fitness
♦ Strength fitness
♦ Flexibility

Cardiorespiratory Fitness

Cardiorespiratory fitness or steady-rate endurance is defined as fitness for the heart, lungs, and blood vessels. To get heart-pumping benefits, you should engage in aerobic exercise for 20–60 minutes in a continuous time frame three days a week or an intermittent minimum of three 10-minute bouts accumulated throughout the day at least three times a week.

Aerobic exercise (often called simply *cardio*), which includes running, walking, cycling, swimming, using cardio-machines, or participating in an aerobics class, may lower your risk of heart disease, diabetes, and cancer. But if you goal is to shed a few pounds, you may need to sweat it out for no less than 60 minutes a day, according to a fairly new study by The Institute of Medicine.

The duration (length) of your cardio is vital to achieving your goals whether they're weight loss or disease prevention. To reach your duration goal, you can, for example, control your intensity level or how hard you work out. Let's say that your fitness goal is disease prevention. A 20–60 minute workout of moderate aerobic exercise three days a week has been proven to help stave off some of today's most debilitating diseases. If your goal is weight loss or weight maintenance, then you may need to sweat it out longer at a lower intensity so you can physically sustain a cardio workout for 60 minutes each day.

On the Ball

A study published by the Institute of Medicine (IOM) reported that to lose weight you must engage in aerobic exercise for 60 minutes every day at a moderate intensity level such as walking to a slow jog. The duration of physical activity, according to the report, is necessary in the prevention of weight gain as well as achieving full health benefits from activity. Previous physical activity recommendations from the U.S. Surgeon General, the American College of Sports Medicine (ACSM), the Center for Disease Control (CDC), and the National Institute of Health stated that you must engage in 20 minutes of cardio, three to four times a week to achieve health benefits. Of course, this report stirred plenty of controversy and confusion! What it means is this: While the IOM report underscores the numerous health benefits that can be obtained from three 10-minute walks a day, it clearly states exercise guidelines for weight loss, and previous physical activity recommendations were for disease prevention only.

Strength

Strength is the foundation for muscular fitness. It includes the ability to lift a heavy object and the ability to repeatedly use a muscle, or muscular endurance. A balanced fitness formula requires both.

As you get older, muscles lose mass. This loss also means a decrease in balance, flexibility, and coordination. Strength is the foundation of these elements of fitness, which is why resistance training is an integral part of fitness. Best of all, muscle is active tissue. Having good muscle strength plays a vital role in regulating your metabolism—the more muscles you have the more fat you burn.

ACSM guidelines recommend strength training, which includes 8–10 exercises of each major muscle group, two to three days a week.

Flexibility

The last element of fitness is flexibility. As with resistance training, ACSM recommends stretching all major muscle groups at least two to three days a week. Stretching falls under two categories: static and dynamic. Static stretching holds a stretch for a certain period of time such as yoga; where as, dynamic stretching moves your body through a stretch, such as Pilates.

If you don't stretch, your muscles lose length. Compounding the problem is age. We all lose flexibility as the years add on. A simple every day task such as bending down to pick something up can become a struggle, which diminishes quality of life.

Loss of flexibility can disturb the proper balance between different muscles in your body, which can affect your posture, leave you miserable with numbing pain, or make you susceptible to an injury.

On the Ball

A personal trainer, health club, or perhaps your doctor can test you in any of the elements of fitness: cardiorespiratory fitness, strength, body fat composition, and flexibility. Based on the results, you can set goals and then continually monitor your progress so that you can work toward a balanced body.

The Fat Factor

The fact is you can be thin with too much fat on you or heavy but healthy. Testing your body composition, therefore, is a more accurate method in measuring the ratio of fat to lean muscle in your body. We all know that it's not healthy to be obese. The dangers are well documented: high blood pressure, type 2 diabetes, heart disease, arthritis … the list goes on! Measuring your body fat can tell you how much fat you're carrying so that you can set fitness goals from that information.

Don't depend on the scale to tell you what's happening in your body. Those numbers can be down right depressing and not always kind. But the good news is that lean muscle is denser and weighs more than fat, which can explain why you've actually gained weight while exercising. In other words, healthy and heavy may not be such a bad thing. Best of all, muscles burn fat and the more muscle you have the more calories you'll burn.

Ball Fitness

Can a ball build fitness? The short answer is yes! The long answers are listed below.

You can use the ball to strength train. In just about every ball exercise, you coordinate your entire musculature to achieve more balance and strength. Ball workouts adapt an integrated approach to training and are functional because within any given exercise you strengthen multiple muscles. This is how your muscles work in your real life. Can you think of an every day move that requires both balance and strength? How about walking up a flight of stairs while carrying bags of groceries?

You can use the ball to lengthen your muscles. Because the ball is big and round, it makes an excellent prop to modify or increase a stretch.

You can use the ball to enhance your cardio. However, in this book the ball is not used as a cardio conditioner. But many gyms offer a cardio class that combines strength and cardio training on the ball, such as a circuit class. To get a balanced body, please do some cardio, such as walking, running, or taking an aerobics class, and following the ACSM guidelines.

The ball can alter your fat to lean ratio in favor of lean. Because strengthening tones your muscles, you can look forward to losing the poochy belly and those dimples around your hips and thighs. You might even see visible body results faster because you're asking your muscles to do more in each exercise—can you imagine the mega-calories used during an entire ball workout?

The Ball and Beyond

Beyond the traditional "big 3," there are other fitness elements of the ball that are equally important to your life's performance, falling under the term functional fitness: balance, postural or core strength, and body sense, interrelating with posture, strength, and proper body alignment. They're not necessarily the "big 3," but each element moves you through your day. When these skills are sharp, your body performs like a lean, mean, very smart machine.

Balance Training

Balance and muscle contraction are an integral part of physical movement. Balance provides the foundation for movement and because the ball creates both strength and balance challenges in an integrated manner, your overall quality of

movement improves. You must instinctively learn how to stabilize your body on the ball, and, therefore, you develop a sense of where your body is at that moment. Simultaneously, you're asking your mind and muscles to coordinate, which improves your balance and coordination skills.

Postural Training

Sitting on the ball requires an orchestra of middle muscles to help stabilize and support your spine: Strong postural muscles provide a support system for your trunk and help move it through its natural movements such as flexion, extension, and rotation. Strong postural muscles help stabilize your pelvis and shoulders so that injury-prone areas such as the lower back and shoulder joints stay healthy. Strong postural muscles can reduce the workload for your limbs as you learn to tap into your body source of power—your core! And finally, strong postural muscles provide a support system for good posture.

On the Ball

Strong abdominal muscles (often called abdominals or just abs) may lead you to the fountain of youth! A recent Canadian study, published by the *Journal of Medicine and Science in Sports and Exercise,* found that participants with weak abs experienced a higher death rate than those with strong abdominals. Peter T. Katzmarzyk, Ph.D., of York University in Ontario, co-authored the study and found the results perplexing, but offered a possible reason. "Skeletal muscle is a major storage site for glucose in the body. It may be that abdominal musculature endurance is a marker for glucose metabolism which helps protect against many chronic diseases, such as Type 2 diabetes and heart disease."

If, however, your middle muscles are weak, your posture may not be on par. As a result, keeping the ball steady underneath you may be a little challenging. This instant feedback helps you make postural improvement while sitting on the ball and, therefore, begins to strengthen these muscles. So, eventually, your posture will improve, your spine will have vital protection and support, your body awareness will heighten as you learn the difference between good and bad alignment, and your mind and muscles will get stronger as they instinctively work together to keep you sitting tall on the ball—and in life (see Chapter 3).

Body Sense Training

Ball training requires an integrated response from your mind and muscles. As the ball rolls, it's your brain that must involuntarily figure out a way to keep you sitting on the ball and then transmit that information to your muscles so you stay balanced on the ball. This body sense eventually carries over to your everyday life: How do you know how to ride a bike after years of not riding one? How do you know instinctively to swerve to avoid a car accident? How do you catch yourself from falling on a wet surface? It's called *proprioception*, which is a sixth sense telling you how to react within a split second in a crisis situation or in a moment in your life.

Ball exercises train your body and brain to be aware of your body's whereabouts and how each body part is positioned spatially—within that moment—hence proprioception. We all possess some degree of body sense or proprioception; however, ball training can hone this skill, improving your reaction time in the event of a fall or slip. Proprioception can be strengthened just like any other fitness element. Use it or lose it!

Good balance requires a joint effort among your inner ears, eyes, spine, and numerous muscles to coordinate this entire proprioception process. Furthermore, good posture and plenty of strength also play a major role in the development of balance. All of these elements are interrelated and when you're effectively trained in these areas, your body performs at its peak. The ball, then, is the perfect piece of equipment to challenge your balance, strengthen your postural strength, and hone your body sense.

Your mind controls your muscles, but you're only as strong as your muscles. Your mind and muscles comprise a carefully balanced system. Much of what you'll do on the ball fine-tunes this system to make all movement a little safer while you get a balanced ball body.

Body Ball Language

Proprioception is having a certain body sense of where the body is in its space. Ball training strengthens proprioception and enhances your brain to body connection.

On the Ball

Ball training forces you to maintain your center of gravity on the ball, which is dynamic and forever changing. This improves your balance skills, which is mind and muscle coordination.

On or Off the Ball

Optimal health requires fitness, but that's only half the equation. Reducing your stress, deepening your sleep, and enhancing your outlook on life can also play a part in achieving good health. Your get so much more out of life when you feel good! Although the ball is a versatile piece of equipment, you must do your part to cultivate a healthy lifestyle. Time spent reflecting on how you feel and listening to your body are equally important to achieving body tone. To get a happier and healthier life, you may want to consider these other aspects of a healthy lifestyle:

◆ Eat a balanced diet consisting of plenty of proteins, hearty multi-grain carbohydrates, good oils including olive oil, plus colorful plates of food, which include a lot of fruits and vegetables.

◆ Drink a lot of water, about a half gallon of water each day, especially if you're exercising every day. Not only does your skin love it, it helps purify toxins from your body.

◆ Get plenty of sleep each night so you don't compromise the quality of your life and your workouts, which can help you sleep better in the first place.

◆ Put a little more weekend in your week, taking time to rest, relax, and renew.

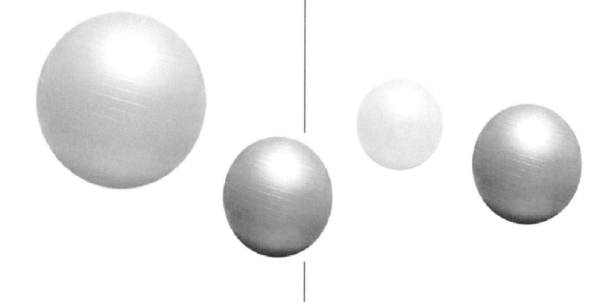

The Least You Need to Know

◆ Fitness improves your overall health; it's the ability to live your life so you have enough energy to meet your day-to-day demands with energy to spare.

◆ According to The American College of Sports Medicine (ACSM), fitness is defined as: cardiorespiratory fitness, strength, flexibility, and body composition.

◆ Because the ball coordinates your entire musculature to achieve more balance and strength, these workouts call for multiple muscle groups to work together like you use them in real life situations.

◆ Ball training hones your balance, strengthens your postural muscles, and sharpens your body's senses as they interrelate to posture and proper body alignment.

In This Chapter

- ◆ Posture performance
- ◆ Hold yourself high on the ball
- ◆ Anatomy in-depth
- ◆ A spine-chilling workout

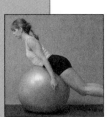
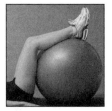
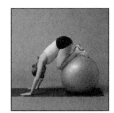
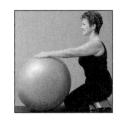
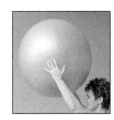
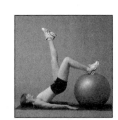

Chapter 3

Body Ball Wisdom

What's the quickest way to look years younger and pounds thinner? Perfect your posture. Read on to learn about posture, the middle muscles that keep you standing tall, and why posture is so important.

Posture Performance (the Truth)

The things we do everyday can chip away at our good posture. We work long hours twisting and turning our spine in all kinds of positions. We slouch to talk on the phone. We slump over daily reports. We scrunch over our computers. And then wonder, "Hmmm, why are my shoulders round? Am I shorter? Why can't I lose thickness around my waist? Why am I so stiff?"

Can the ball help? You bet! Proper alignment is a must for you to do the exercises correctly; otherwise, you might fall off the ball. The natural urge not to fall keeps you sitting tall with good alignment, trains your mind as to what good posture feels like, and strengthens your muscles to support good posture.

Knowing a little about these muscles is the first step in the development of good posture, and it provides an opportunity for you to make some corrections in your body, whether exercising or sitting on the couch. After all, isn't that the perfect definition of fitness—enhancing your life's performance?

So what's *good posture*? Here's the short answer: good body alignment. And here's the long answer: Good posture means aligning your body as a whole and its body parts individually so they can perform an action with maximum efficiency and minimum wear on the body. To do this, you need a combination of core strength, balance, coordination, and body awareness—all elements of functional fitness (see Chapter 2). Training on the ball improves these areas of fitness, and you'll walk away with a better sense of knowing how to hold yourself. The truth is that posture plays a major roll in keeping you healthy. Not only will you protect your back from a lifetime of aches and pains, you'll radiate confidence. The following also come with good posture:

◆ You'll look ten pounds lighter, and your waistline shrinks in inches.

◆ You'll prevent back pain as a result of poor posture.

◆ You'll look inches taller.

◆ You'll have more energy as your breathing capacity improves.

Body Ball Language

Good posture means aligning your body as a whole and its parts individually so they can perform an action with maximum efficiency and minimum wear on the body.

Back Basics

Your spine is your anatomical life support; it adds up to a column of spinal bones or vertebrae that allow you to move, and it is the home of your life force—the spinal cord. An unhealthy spine can leave you miserable with pain or lower your resistance to diseases.

What keeps you from collapsing is an interrelated complex system of bone, ligaments, tendons, cartilage, discs, nerves, and muscles. When efficient, these elements align your spine with precise musculoskeletal integrity. But an injury can happen at any given moment to any of these systems. And because your body is a closed chain system, a breakdown to any component can cause a system-wide meltdown. When one part fails another part must overcompensate to keep your body functional.

The good news is that you can greatly reduce your chances of a system-wide meltdown by having good posture and strong and supple postural muscles.

Navigating Neutral

Much of what you do on the ball is strengthen the muscles that support your spine to maintain good alignment. Notice that your spine is not straight, it has three natural curves. Feel free to look in the mirror and evaluate the health of your spine as you read about its curves:

◆ The first curve creates an arch between the base of your neck and the upper back; it's called your cervical curve and actually begins deep between your ears and then travels down your spine making up the first seven vertebrae, C1–C7.

◆ As you travel down your spine, you may notice a slight hump in the middle of your back. That's your thoracic curve which consists of 12 vertebrae, T1–T12.

◆ Keep going, and you may notice a slight arch between the area of your spine and pelvis. This low curve is your lumbar spine, which adds up to only 5 vertebrae, L1–L5. Your lower back is most vulnerable to pain because the majority of body weight is held in this area. Slouching, for example, puts tremendous pressure on your lumbar vertebrae.

◆ Attached to the lower lumbar are five sacral vertebrae (S1–S5) fused together as one flat bone of your buttocks; it's called the sacrum.

◆ And finally, the coccygeal vertebrae are nonmovable bones consisting of four vertebrae acting as one unit; it's your tailbone.

On the Ball

Research shows that good posture projects health, vitality, and confidence; whereas, hunching suggests weakness, gloom, and self-doubt.

To decrease risk of injury while training on the ball, you'll keep these bones in their proper place or a *neutral spine position*. A neutral spine lessens your chances of injury because this position places the least amount of stress on your body. If your spine is aligned, so, too, are your ligaments, tendons, muscles, and discs. This way, all systems operate at peak performance because the whole body is under the least amount of stress.

Body Ball Language

Neutral spine position aligns the natural curves of your spine so all systems can operate with peak performance because the whole body is under the least amount of stress.

Remember, your spine is only functional with the help of an interrelated system depending on one another. If one system fails, another must pick up slack, which increases your chances of wear and tear on that particular body part. Worse yet, overuse sets off a downward spiral of pain. Neutral, however, trains your trunk in an optimal position so as not to stress this entire system. If you don't train in a neutral spine position, you risk strengthening the muscles incorrectly and reinforcing poor alignment. But by strengthening your muscles in a neutral position, you're also building a strong support system for your frame, and, eventually, you'll be able to distinguish between bad posture and good posture.

Two areas of your body directly influence what your spine is doing: the hip-pelvis and shoulder-scapula areas. Collectively, these two areas of your body add up to the many muscles and bones that attach the limbs to your spine and help to establish a neutral spine. Therefore, these complexes must remain stable or neutral before any movement can begin to help reduce any excessive stress to your body.

Pelvis Perfection

Because the hip-pelvis complex directly influences your spine's position, it's vitally important that you exercise or stretch with your pelvis in a stable (neutral) position. When you train with a stable *pelvis*, you strengthen your abdominals to support your lower back, helping to relieve its workload. Most people feel that their lower backs are weak when in fact their backs are stressed. Part of the problem is not having a support system in place, which includes strong abdominals.

Finding a neutral pelvis is a little tricky; it's not mashing your back into the floor nor is it an exaggerated arch. Neutral is right in the middle of those two extreme positions. Here's a trick to finding neutral: Imagine that your pelvis is a bowl filled to the brim with water. You must find a position that keeps the water in place—hence, a neutral pelvis. Overarching your lumbar spine spills the water in front of your thighs; whereas, a flat lumbar spine trickles the water down the back of your legs. Experiment—move your pelvis through these positions to find neutral.

Every exercise and stretch calls for a stable pelvis, so the following are a few tips on how to navigate neutral. Try this exercise on the floor before attempting it on the ball where it becomes more challenging.

1. Lie on the floor with your knees bent.
2. Place the right palm of your hand on the area between your hip bone and pubic bone.
3. Move your pelvis so your lower back mashes to the floor. Notice that your fingertips rise as your pubic bone does.
4. Now, move your pelvis the other direction so that your lower back arches. This time, the palm of your hand will rise and send your pubic bone to the floor.
5. After moving through these extreme positions, end up in a stable pelvis. That's when your hand rests evenly between those two bony points; it's okay if you have a little arch in your back, but nothing extreme.

Shoulder Smarts

On your upper spine floats a pair of winged-bones called shoulder blades or scapulae. These bones directly influence the position of your shoulders and are part of a complex of bones and muscles that attach your arms to your spine. Simply put, just like your pelvis influences your lower spine's position, these bones influence what your upper spine is doing.

Your goal is to learn how to stabilize your shoulder blades so your shoulders remain in their place. Why is this important? Because most people walk around in a constant state of shoulder shrugs. Chronic shoulder elevation is the plague of our stressed out society. So the first step is to be aware of how you hold your shoulders and then you can begin to build a support system to ensure proper alignment.

Try this: Inhale to lift your shoulders to your ears and then slightly back. Exhale to float your shoulder blades down your back. Notice that sliding them into place also depresses your shoulders—this is called shoulder-scapula stabilization.

Only when your shoulder girdle is stable can you preserve the integrity of your upper spine and strengthen its support system (muscles) correctly to lessen your risk of injury and poor posture. To help slide your shoulder blades into their pockets, try this mini-exercise. You'll need a hand towel.

1. Sit on the floor in a comfortable position.
2. Place a towel in your hands and then lift your arms over your head.
3. Lift your shoulders to your ears.
4. Now, pull on both ends of the towel to drop your shoulders and slide your shoulder blades down your back.
5. Hold this isometric contraction to train your mind and muscles to ensure proper activation of the shoulder-scapular area.

Middle Muscles That Matter

Strengthening your postural muscles not only helps establish a support system for your pelvis and shoulders, but a strong middle improves your posture and protects your back from injury. Your trunk is arranged in several layers of overlapping muscles. Some provide brace-like support for your spine, whereas other muscles help move it. Some muscles are common while others are obscure yet equally important to your spine's health—and your good looks.

Let's take a look at your middle muscles, from the deepest to the most superficial ones. The transversus abdominis or transverse is the deepest of all of your abdominal muscles and sits deep in your trunk. Because of its anatomical wrap around the spine, the transverse stabilizes your spine as it contracts, forming a deep girdle of spinal support by pulling your abdominal wall near your spine. Your goal is to tap

into its strength in every exercise for spinal protection and to give you a little extra oomph. If done correctly, you feel your belly button pull in toward your spine as if a belt tightens around your waist.

The multifidus also helps provide spinal support; it, on the other hand, is a posterior muscle spanning three layers deep and runs the length of your spine, from the sacrum to the cervical vertebrae. And finally, there are your pelvic floor muscles that also assist in keeping your spine stable. The pelvic floors span five layers deep to cross through the bottom of the pelvis, from the pubic bone to the coccyx (anus)—imagine a hammock—and from butt bone to butt bone (you sit on these bones). Collectively, these muscles work in harmony to play a major roll in providing spinal stability.

On the Ball

Your trunk muscles are arranged in several layers from the deepest to the most superficial. Three deep muscles, the transverse, multifidus, and pelvic floors, co-contract to support your spine and protect it.

Sitting on top of your transverse are the abdominal obliques:

◆ The internal oblique sit on top of the transverse, originate on the pelvis, and insert on the lower ribs.

◆ The external obliques sit on top of the internal obliques, originate on the lower ribs, and insert on the pelvis. They form an "X" across the abdomen to provide trunk support and assist in rotation. They bend sideways at the waist.

◆ The rectus abdominis is the most superficial muscle. It runs from the pubic bone to breastbone so that you can bend forward.

Now, let's change directions. The most common and often overworked group of back muscles is called erector spinae. These muscles form a broad band around your vertebrae and are superficial to the multifidus. The main action of these muscles is to bend your spine backward—referred to as spinal extension. The multifidus, on the other hand, although it has some extension components, works primarily to facilitate core stabilization in the neutral spine position.

Continue up your back and you'll find many more amazing muscles. Some provide upper back support while others move and stabilize your shoulder blades, which directly influence the position of your shoulders. There are four muscles acting on your shoulder blades:

◆ The rhomboids rest between your shoulder blades to help open and close them.

◆ The trapezius or traps form a diamond shape on your back, extending from the base of your skull to the back part of your shoulders and down the middle of your back, and they help lower and lift your shoulder blades and help depress your shoulders.

◆ And there's a tiny muscle that also helps stabilize your shoulder blades; it's called the serratus anterior. This muscle stretches from your lateral rib cage and has dual responsibilities. Not only does it help in stabilizing your shoulder blades, it also assists in respiration.

◆ And finally there's a very important back muscle you should be aware of, latissimus dorsi. Your lats are a broad and superficial back muscle, wrapping from your sacrum to your front ribs. By wrapping from front to back, this muscle helps preserve the structural integrity of your trunk during various movements.

Maintaining trunk integrity is so much easier when these muscles are strong. The good news is you don't have to set out to work your middle because of the dynamic nature of the ball; it does it for you! In every exercise you'll challenge and strengthen your middle muscles while testing your steadiness on the ball. And yet there's an added bonus—love handle–free and fabulous abs!

Hippity-Hop or Hippity-Flop?

Now that you're ready and raring to get on the ball, keep in mind that the ball can be both functional and spine-chilling. What's most appealing about the fitness ball is also scary— you can exercise in a variety of positions because it lifts you off the floor. So your workout doesn't turn hippity-flop, sending you to floor, here are a few safety ball guidelines:

◆ Practice good form because it will help you stay afloat.

◆ Alternate your base of support depending on your physical ability. For example, when sitting on the ball, you can lessen the intensity by widening your legs. Or you can increase the intensity by bringing your knees closer together, narrowing your base of support.

◆ Alter your center of gravity and the degree of difficulty will change. By having the majority of your body off the ball, the exercise becomes more difficult. In other words, the farther your limbs are away from the ball, the harder your postural muscles must work to stabilize you on the ball. If you keep your body close to the ball, the exercise level decreases in intensity.

◆ Increase your body's workload by adding dumbbell weights. As your body gets stronger, dumbbell weights can keep muscles challenged. (You don't have to work with weights depending on your fitness level.)

◆ Lift your limbs to change your base of support. To increase the intensity level of an exercise, you can lift your arm or your leg depending on the exercise.

Before You Begin

These ball workouts add a cross-training element to your existing fitness formula or you can specifically design your week around them. As with any exercise program, there is risk. Try your very best to work out with good form and common sense. Below are some pitfalls to be aware of when exercising:

◆ Don't blow off your warm-up! Muscles need to warm-up gradually—sending them into a muscle shock could cause injury.

◆ Your muscles must cool down as well because blood goes to the working muscles. If you just stop, you may experience some lightheadedness as the muscles are still pulled to your working muscles. Take five minutes to allow your body to cool down.

◆ Don't jerk or swing your weights into position. Stabilize your spine and use muscle not momentum.

◆ Perform a mental checklist of good posture before starting any exercise.

◆ Don't use too much weight.

◆ Set realistic exercise goals for yourself especially if you're a first timer. Start small and then work up to more lofty exercise goals; otherwise, you may set yourself up for failure.

◆ Think quality versus quantity.

◆ Drink a lot of water. If you're thirsty, it's too late.

◆ Variety keeps your muscles from getting bored and you as well so cross train. Don't get stuck in a rut.

The Least You Need to Know

◆ Most minor back pain is preventable with a well-balanced exercise program that includes strengthening the postural muscles.

◆ Your goal is to align your spine so that its three natural curves remain in a neutral position, hence the term neutral spine.

◆ Good alignment means that your body as a whole and its parts individually are aligned in a position where they can perform with maximum efficiency with minimum wear on the body.

◆ Much of what you do on the ball strengthens the middle muscles that support the spine so that you work toward perfect posture.

In This Part

4 Beginner Ball Bliss

5 The Body Ball Makeover

6 Mind-Body Ball Blitz

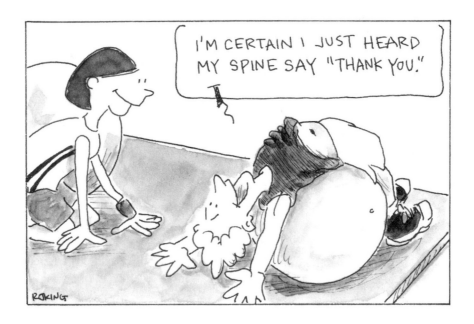

Part 2

Get Your Best Ball Body

In Chapter 4, I demonstrate a variety of exercises that strengthen your spine, giving you postural stability, so that you can stay on the ball. You can then move to the total body strength moves in Chapter 5, in which you move your arms and legs, challenging your stability on the ball even more. With your new strength, you can advance to the most challenging workout, in Chapter 6, where each exercise calls for multiple muscles and balance challenges. Each workout varies in intensity so you can begin your ball journey or use these exercises to keep your mind and muscles challenged for quite some time.

In This Chapter

- ◆ Ball basics
- ◆ Build postural strength and stability
- ◆ Posture perfection
- ◆ Tap into your internal power

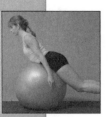
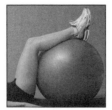
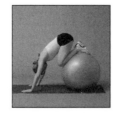
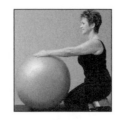
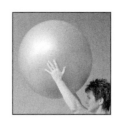
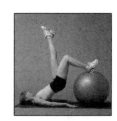

Chapter 4

Beginner Ball Bliss

Let's start with nine basic ball exercises that form the backbone of most ball workouts (whether you're in the gym or taking a group exercise class). Because you'll rock 'n' roll on a ball, this workout develops postural stability and strength by uncovering your abs and back muscles. You'll first instinctively train your body to stay on the ball and then develop plenty of strength so you really do.

Let's begin by tapping your internal power which is a source of strength for your spine. Of course, this strength keeps you on the ball, too.

Ball Basics: Beginner Exercises

To make your fitness workout complete, pick a low intensity cardio workout and do it for 20–30 minutes. A leisure walk or moderate workout on a cardio machine is fine. Keep it light, though, so you have enough energy for this ball workout. Keep at this routine for about six to eight weeks or until you feel confident to advance to the next chapter. You won't need any props, just your ball and a mat.

This postural workout is just that—a way for you to tap into postural muscles. To help you move in and out of these postural exercises, you'll use your breath, especially a lengthened exhalation to build strength in the stabilizing muscles of your spine, so read the directions carefully and follow the specific breathing requirements for each exercise. If you need more of a physical challenge, try three sets of each exercise. Do this workout two to three times a week as part of a strength training routine.

Do two sets of each of the following exercises, which are the subject of this chapter:

◆ Seated ball postural exercises (neutral, lateral rocks with hip circles, and leg and arm raises)

◆ Squat off the ball (transition)

◆ Walk down the ball (transition)

◆ Abdominal ball curls

◆ Supine ball bridge

◆ Spinal ball extension

◆ Drape over the ball

◆ Cross ball extension

◆ Stationary ball plank

◆ Ball bridge on the floor

On the Ball

Sitting on the ball stimulates deep abdominal and back muscles; it's essential to begin by strengthening these muscles because they provide stability for your spine. To tap into your internal power, you use your breath. A deep exhalation pulls your belly in (try coughing to feel this contraction) and triggers your transverse and the other spine stabilizing muscles. In all exercises, focus on your breath, specifically your exhalation.

Seated Ball Postural Exercises: Finding a Neutral Spine on the Ball

Why it works: Sitting on the ball is harder than you may think. This active work requires that you engage your stabilizing muscles and then maintain the activation so that these muscles support your spine.

While sitting on the ball, you'll move in and out of several positions and then return to a neutral spine. This exercise increases spinal mobility, develops lumbar and pelvic awareness, trains you to recognize what good posture feels like and warms up your lumbar spine.

Start/Finish Position

1. Sit on the top of your ball with your knees hip-width apart, feet parallel and firmly grounded to the floor.

2. Ground your sitting bones, which are located directly under the cheeky portion of your bottom.

3. Inhale to roll your shoulders up to your ears and slightly back and then draw your shoulder blades down your back.

4. Lift your belly button up and in under your rib cage toward your spine.

5. Pay attention to your spinal curves as they maintain a stable (neutral) spine.

6. Place your hands on your thighs.

7. Take several deep breaths, focusing on exhalation to activate your deep stabilizing muscles.

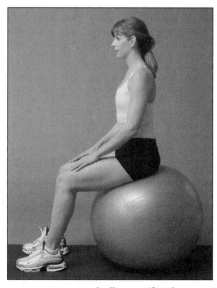

Sitting on ball, start/finish.

Movement One

This pelvic tilt position flattens your lumbar spine and pulls your navel deeper to your spine.

8. Inhale to grow tall in your spine.
9. Exhale to tip your pubic bone to the ceiling, and let the ball roll slightly forward.
10. Return to a neutral spine.

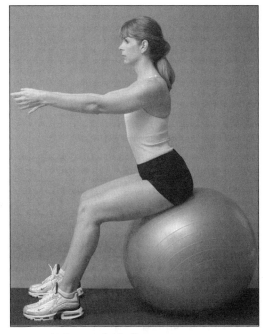

Sitting on the ball, movement two.

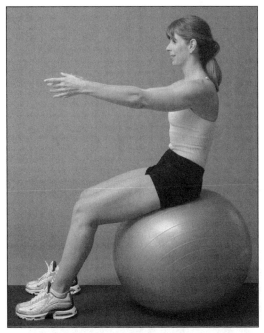

Sitting on the ball, movement one.

Movement Two

This anterior tilt position creates an arch in your lumbar spine.

11. Inhale to grow tall in your spine.
12. Exhale to move your pubic bone to the floor, and let the ball roll slightly behind you.
13. Return to a neutral spine.

Balancing Ball Tips

◆ You're engaging your middle muscles in these exercises, so focus on them.

◆ Lengthen through the top of your head, creating a long neck and spine.

◆ Don't force the movement; use your abdominal muscles to move the bones of your pelvis.

◆ Maintain the natural curves of your spine while sitting on the ball.

◆ Specifically pay attention to your pelvis. Remember, neutral pelvis is when your pubic bone and hip bones are in the same line. If you need a review, turn to Chapter 3.

◆ Maintain upper spine stability by drawing your shoulder blades down your back, which will prevent your shoulders from lifting to your ears.

◆ If you need less of a challenge, then put your hands on your thighs to help you balance.

◆ Keep in mind that these exercises warm up the spine, so you'll do them first in all of the workouts to come.

Seated Ball Postural Exercises: Ball Rocking

Why it works: This exercise engages your postural muscles while strengthening and stretching many obscure muscles of your lower back and waist—such as your abdominal obliques. Remember, your obliques cross your abdomen diagonally to help provide trunk support. After moving from side-to-side, return to a stable spine and complete five to eight circles and then reverse the direction to enhance your pelvic awareness and warm up your lumbar spine.

Start/Finish Position

1. Sit on the center of your ball with your knees hip-width apart, feet parallel and firmly grounded to the floor.
2. Place your hands on your thighs.
3. Relax your shoulders.

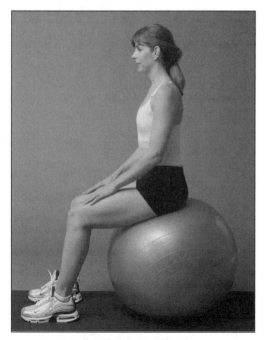

Ball rocking, start/finish.

Movement One

4. Shift your pelvis to the right so that the ball rolls with you.
5. As the bones of your pelvis move from side to side, activate your abdominals, focusing on your waist muscles.

   (Try this exercise with your hands on your thighs, but if you would like more core challenge, raise your arms as you see in the following figure.)

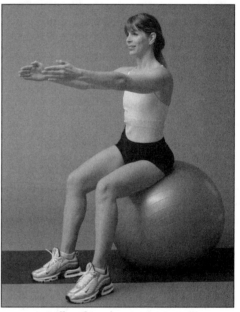

Ball rocking, movement one.

Movement Two

6. Now shift your pelvis to the left so that the ball rolls with you.

   (Try this exercise with your hands on your thighs, but if you would like more core challenge, raise your arms as you see in the following figure.)

7. Return to a neutral spine.

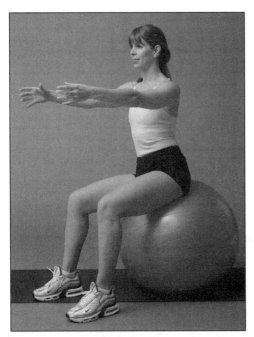

Ball rocking, movement two.

On the Ball

There are three primary muscles that stabilize your spine: transverse (abdominal), multifidus (back muscle), and pelvic floors. And yet, there are a variety of muscles that support your trunk. The most recognized ones are the abdominal obliques and rectus abdominus, and the back muscles that support your trunk are the erector spinae and latissimus dorsi.

Balancing Ball Tips

◆ You're engaging your middle muscles in these exercises, so focus on them.

◆ Lengthen through the top of your head, creating a long neck and spine.

◆ Don't force the movement; use your abdominal muscles to move the bones of your pelvis.

◆ Maintain the natural curves of your spine while sitting on the ball.

◆ Specifically pay attention to your pelvis. Remember, neutral pelvis is when your pubic bone and hip bones are in the same line. If you need a review, turn to Chapter 3.

◆ Maintain upper spine stability by drawing your shoulder blades down your back, which will prevent your shoulders from lifting to your ears.

◆ If you feel too wobbly on the ball, then put your hands on your thighs during the actual exercise.

◆ Keep in mind that these exercises warm up the spine, so you'll do them first in all of the workouts to come.

Ball Blowout

If you feel very unsteady on the ball, place the ball against the wall until you feel more secure. Remember, there's no rush!

Seated Ball Postural Exercises: Leg and Arm Raises

Why it works: This exercise strengthens your postural muscles and improves your pelvic awareness as you lift your legs and arms. These exercises increase in intensity because you learn how to maintain a stable spine while raising your legs and arms. Take your time here!

Start/Finish Position

1. Sit on the center of your ball with your knees hip-width apart, feet parallel and firmly grounded to the floor. Your hands are on your thighs to begin this exercise. When ready lower your arms by your sides to place your fingertips on the ball to help keep the ball steady.

2. Slide your shoulder blades down your back to stabilize your shoulder girdle and help activate the muscles of your upper back.

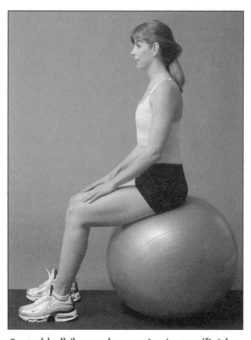

Seated ball (leg and arm raises), start/finish.

Movement One

3. Ground your right foot firmly to floor.

4. With a stable pelvis, lift your left leg. Your fingertips may touch the ball to help stabilize you. Sustain this position for five to eight breaths, focusing on a stable pelvis.

5. Lift the opposite leg. If lifting your legs is too challenging, then stop here.

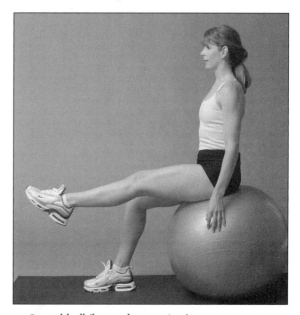

Seated ball (leg and arm raises), movement one.

Movement Two

6. This time, lift your left leg and right arm at the same time.

7. Sustain this position for five to eight breaths.

8. Repeat to opposite arm and leg.

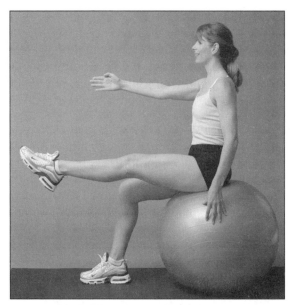

Seated ball (leg and arm raises), movement two.

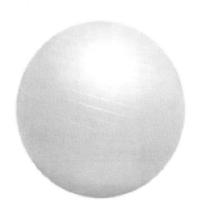

On the Ball _____

If you would like to increase the balance challenge, try doing these exercises with your eyes closed.

Balancing Ball Tips

◆ To keep yourself steady, focus on exhaling to engage your stabilizing spine muscles, which helps steady your trunk.

◆ As you lift your leg off the floor, your pelvis may want to shift forward into a flat back position. This could be a sign of hamstring tightness. Use your exhalation to help keep your pelvis stable. But if you feel too wobbly, don't lift your leg. You'll have an opportunity to stretch your hamstrings in Chapter 10.

◆ If you feel really wobbly, don't lift your leg off the ground very high. Test the waters by keeping your big toe on the floor.

◆ Don't forget to lengthen through the top of your head, think tall.

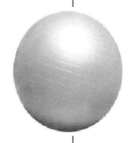

Squat off the Ball

Why it works: Squat off the ball is not really an exercise but rather a lesson in how to get on and off the ball. This strength carries over to your everyday life. After all, good strength in your legs along with proper form can help you get out of a stationary chair safely.

Start/Finish Position

1. Sit on the center of your ball with your knees hip-width apart, feet parallel and firmly grounded to the floor.
2. Raise your arms so they are in front of you and parallel to the floor.
3. Relax your shoulders.

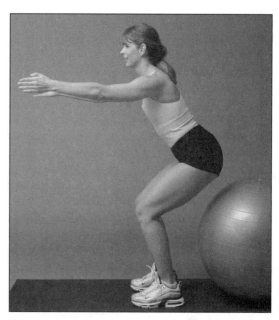

Squat off the ball, movement one.

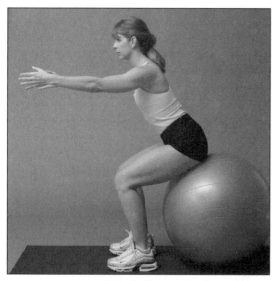

Squat off the ball, start/finish.

Movement

4. From a sitting position, bend your knees, gently rock forward to lift your butt off the ball into a squat position. Hold this squat for five to eight breaths.
5. Carefully sit back down on the ball.
6. Repeat three to five times.

Balancing Ball Tips

◆ Be careful. The ball may roll out from underneath you as you squat off the ball.

◆ Use the strength of your legs and abdominals to lift you off the ball and to hold the squat. Don't push or strain your lower back.

◆ Don't extend your knees past your toes. Try aligning your knees between your second and third toes and place the majority of your body weight in your heels.

◆ If this squat is too hard, try placing your hands on your thighs.

◆ You can always place the ball against the wall, if you find this exercise difficult.

Ball Blowout

Maintain good alignment: Your ears are over your shoulders, and shoulders are over your hips. Belly button is pulled up and in under your ribs, engaging your trunk muscles to keep your spine stable.

Walking down the Ball

Why it works: Walking down the ball is used as a transition from sitting on the ball to sitting on the floor or somewhere between. Anytime you read "walk down the ball," follow these instructions.

Start/Finish Position

1. Sit on the center of your ball with your knees hip-width apart, feet parallel and firmly grounded to the floor.

2. In one motion, begin to walk your feet away as your arms simulate a walk.

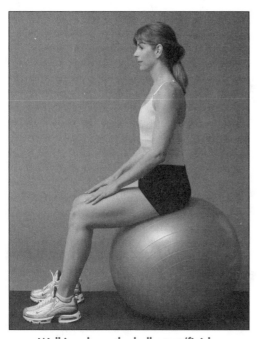

Walking down the ball, start/finish.

Movement

3. Continue walking until your mid-back touches the ball and your bottom is off the ball. The back of your arms may touch the ball.

4. Reverse your walk to sit on the ball.

5. Practice walking down and up three to five times.

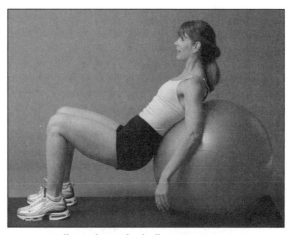

Walking down the ball, movement one.

Balancing Ball Tips

◆ Maintain a neutral pelvis even though your back is supported by the ball.

◆ Your abs are active.

◆ Try holding this squat position to strengthen the muscles in your legs.

◆ If you experience any knee strain, look at how you're tracking your knees. Your knees should not extend past your toes while the bulk of your body weight is placed in your heels.

Abdominal Ball Curls

Why it works: This exercise strengthens your abdominals and legs at the same time. You must learn to stabilize your body on the ball while doing an abdominal curl. Throughout this book, you'll see a variety of abdominal curls varying in degrees of intensity, so you can increase the difficulty factor to keep your abs challenged.

Here's the general rule: The closer your bottom is to the floor, the work load for your abdominals lessens because your legs pick up some of the slack to help stabilize you.

If your bottom stays lifted and more of your torso is on the ball, you increase the abdominal challenge. Experiment here!

Start/Finish Position

1. Sit on the center of your ball with your knees hip-width apart, feet parallel and firmly grounded to the floor.
2. Your arms simulate walking and are active as you begin to "walk down the ball."
3. Drop your bottom toward the floor, using your legs to control your body.
4. Place your hands in a prayer position and place them on your chest.
5. Curl your chin to your chest.
6. Gaze at the wall in front of you.

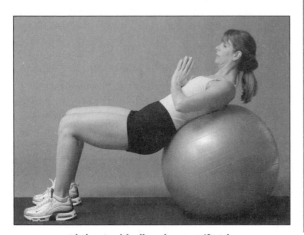

Abdominal ball curls, start/finish.

Movement

7. Inhale to prepare for the exercise.
8. Exhale to lift your shoulders off the ball by about 3 inches.
9. Inhale to return to starting position.

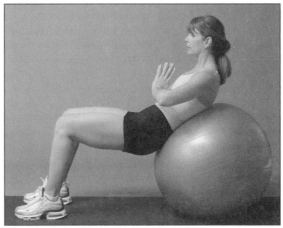

Abdominal ball curls, movement one.

Balancing Ball Tips

◆ As you curl up, exhale and pull your ribs to your hips to engage your abs, specifically your obliques.

◆ Don't look at the ceiling. Instead, gently guide your chin to your chest to avoid overstraining neck muscles and cervical spine.

◆ Exhale as much as you can while curling to engage your transverse.

◆ Don't bounce as you curl up, control your motion especially as you curl down.

◆ Even though your lower back is against the ball, maintain a neutral pelvis.

◆ The ball must not roll, so use your legs.

◆ Don't hold your breath.

Supine Ball Bridge

Why it works: This exercise develops awareness and strength in your pelvis so you can
hold your pelvis and spine stability. A supine
position or faceup on the ball strengthens and
sculpts many muscles of your backside including one of your largest muscles (and hardest to
tone) your gluteus maximus, or buttocks.

Start/Finish Position

1. Sit on the center of your ball with your
   knees hip-width, feet parallel and firmly
   grounded to the floor.
2. Walk down the ball until your upper back
   and neck are on the ball.
3. Place your hands on your thighs.

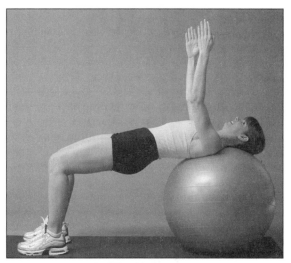

Supine ball bridge, movement one.

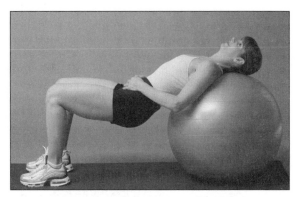

Supine ball bridge, start/finish.

Movement

4. In one motion, lift your hips to the ceiling
   so your thighs are parallel to the floor.
   When steady, raise your arms. Hold this
   bridge for five to eight breaths.
5. Finish by walking up the ball to a sitting
   position.

On the Ball

When working in a supine position or
faceup, remember this: A bowl of soup
must face up!

Balancing Ball Tips

◆ Don't let your head hang off the ball; it
  must be completely on the ball.

◆ Don't lift your chin to the ceiling or force
  your chin to your chest. Maintain a neutral cervical spine.

◆ Align your head, neck, spine, and pelvis in
  a straight line. Your hips are above your
  knees and your knees directly over your
  ankles.

◆ Keep your body weight in your heels to
  feel the work in your butt.

◆ If you feel wobbly, place your fingertips
  on the floor to help stabilize you.

◆ To increase the workload for your thighs,
  place a pillow between them and squeeze it.

◆ Your abdominals are completely engaged
  to keep your bottom from dropping to
  the floor.

◆ Don't lift your hips too high so you don't
  put extra pressure on your lower back.
  Your hip bones are even and in line with
  the rest of your trunk.

◆ Don't place your feet too close to the ball,
  which can strain your knees.

Spinal Ball Extension

Why it works: Spinal extension strengthens the many muscles of your back in a prone or face-down position. To balance your body, you must move the spine in all of its natural movements, which include spinal extension, flexion, and rotation. Spinal extension can be a difficult exercise, so please pay attention to your alignment and listen to your body.

Start/Finish Position

1. Kneel in front of your ball, toes down.
2. Wrap your arms around the ball as you curl your chest, abdomen, and hips over it.
3. Gaze at the floor.

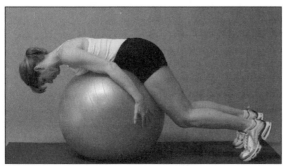

Spinal ball extension, start/finish.

Movement

4. Inhale to lift your chest off the ball, straightening your spine. Lengthen from the top of your head. Keep your head in line with your spine. Hold for three to five breaths.
5. Drape over the ball.

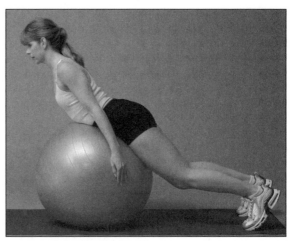

Spinal ball extension, movement one.

Balancing Ball Tips

◆ If you have a lower back injury, please check with your doctor before attempting spinal extension.

◆ Your neck is in line with the whole spine, so gaze at the floor.

◆ It's important to lengthen from the top of your head, so you don't put needless pressure on your lower back.

◆ Keep your hands close to your body.

◆ As you lift into extension, pay particular attention to your shoulders because they may elevate. Slide your shoulder blades down your back to create upper spine and shoulder stability as well.

On the Ball

Training with your face down is called the prone position, which is an ideal position for strengthening the muscles of your backside.

Drape over the Ball

Why it works: Draping over the ball soothes muscles of your back and eases tension in your back. Indulge in this stretch anytime you want because it's a wonderful way to release over-worked back muscles.

Start/Finish Position

1. After spinal extension, stretch your back by rolling the ball under your belly and draping yourself over it.

2. Relax and focus on deep breathing.

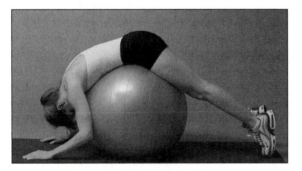

Drape over the ball, start/finish.

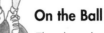

On the Ball

The deep back muscles (many are un-heard of) tend to be arranged in several layers to provide spinal stability and support. Some of the deepest ones consist of small bundles passing from one vertebra to another while others form long superficial layers the length of your spine. The most superficial and overworked back muscle is a bundle of muscles called erector spinae. The main action of this muscle is to extend your spine.

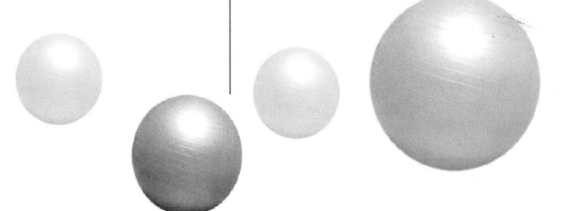

Cross Ball Extension

Why it works: Cross ball extension stretches and strengthens your back muscles while simultaneously teaching you to stabilize your spine against the weight of your limbs.

Start/Finish Position

1. Kneel in front of your ball, toes down.

2. Drape your torso over your ball.

3. Place your hands on the floor in front of your ball and gaze at the floor.

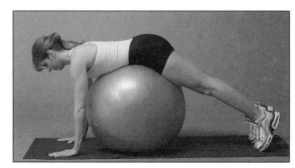

Cross ball extension, start/finish.

Movement

4. Simultaneously, lift your left leg and right arm, pushing through your heel to engage your buttock muscles. Don't lift your chin or drop your head—it should be in line with your spine. Hold this contraction for three to five breaths.

5. Lower your limbs to the floor.

6. Repeat cross extension on opposite side of your body.

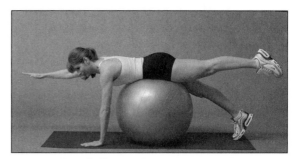

Cross ball extension, movement one.

Balancing Ball Tips

◆ If you have any lower back problems, then you might not want to try this exercise. Please consult your doctor.

◆ Even though your torso is supported by the ball, lift the pit of your belly to the ceiling.

◆ Lift the leg from your heel to activate your glutes and hamstrings.

◆ Don't lift your leg higher than your torso. Keep your hipbones even and maintain a stable pelvis.

Stationary Ball Plank

Why it works: The plank strengthens your shoulders, encourages trunk and shoulder stability, and challenges and strengthens your core. In this plank (you'll see a variety of planks because it's the perfect exercise to build core strength), focus on keeping your shoulders stable.

Start/Finish Position

1. Kneel in front of your ball, rounding your chest, abdomen, and hips over the ball.
2. Place your hands on the floor in front of the ball.

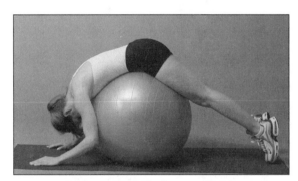

Stationary Ball Plank , start/finish.

Movement

3. Walk your hands out until the ball rolls near your hips; legs are straight.
4. Even though your body is supported by the ball, lift the pit of your belly to the ceiling for trunk support.
5. Place your hands directly under your shoulders (hand placement is vital to the integrity of the exercise).
6. Draw your shoulder blades down your back, creating upper back and shoulder stability.
7. Take five to eight breaths, pulling your navel deeper to your spine with each exhale.
8. After completing your breath work, drape over the ball.

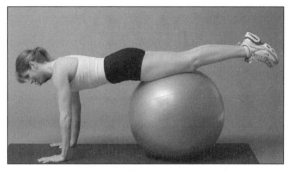

Stationary Ball Plank , movement one.

Balancing Ball Tips

◆ If you have a shoulder, neck, or back injury, check with your doctor before doing this exercise.

◆ Hug your abs to your spine the whole time to stabilize your spine and support your torso so you don't strain your lower back.

◆ Proper hand placement is a must for reinforcing proper upper back alignment plus strengthening your shoulder muscles correctly. Place your hands directly under your shoulders. Slide your shoulder blades down your back to create shoulder and upper back support.

◆ Don't hike your shoulders up to your ears.

◆ If you experience lower back strain, first check your alignment. Perhaps you're not pulling your navel to your spine or your hands are too far from your ball. If the pain persists, stop this exercise.

Ball Blowout

The farther your hands are away from the ball, the harder the plank exercise is. At first, work with the ball close to your hips, and then you can walk your hands out farther to increase the core challenge.

Ball Bridge on the Floor

Why it works: Ball bridge strengthens your trunk muscles, sends awareness to your pelvis, encourages a stable pelvis, and tones the muscles of your backside. Pelvic stability is essential to your spine's health, and therefore, strengthening these muscles can help hold your pelvis steady (aligned), helping to ease the workload of your lower back.

Start/Finish Position

1. Lie on your back with the ball under your knees so it touches the back of your thighs. Your hips and knees are bent at a 90-degree position, arms by your sides.
2. Lengthen your fingertips to your toes.

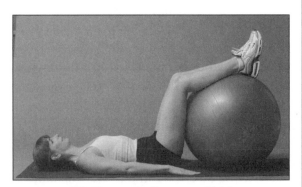

Ball bridge on the floor, start/finish.

Movement One

3. Walk the ball away from your bottom, so it rests against your calves.

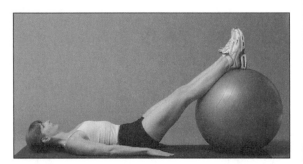

Ball Bridge on the Floor, movement one.

Movement Two

4. In one movement, lift your hips to the ceiling. Hold this Bridge for five to eight breaths.
5. Lower your spine slowly to the floor, as if each bone touches the floor.
6. Roll the ball back under the back of your thighs and relax.

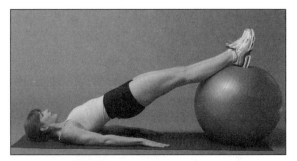

Ball bridge on the floor, movement two.

Balancing Ball Tips

◆ Your shoulders, pelvis, and knees are in one line.
◆ Don't forget to engage your abs, exhaling deeply to pull your belly button to your spine to create core stability.
◆ Initiate the lift by contracting your glutes.
◆ Lower the spine to the floor with control, focusing on each bone of your spine.

Congratulations!

You should feel stronger in your middle including your shoulders and hips. What's most important is that you learned to tap into your internal power source, the stabilizing muscles, for a stable spine. This is body awareness, having the ability to hold your body with proper alignment. As you move to the next chapter, keep in mind that this newly developed trunk strength will help you stay stable on the ball as the workload increases. Good Luck!

The Least You Need to Know

- These exercises strengthen the stabilizing muscles of your trunk.
- Developing spinal stability so your hips and shoulders are aligned helps to strengthen the muscles that support your trunk correctly.
- If you feel very unsteady on the ball, place the ball against the wall until you feel comfortable.
- To maintain good alignment while sitting on the ball, your ears are over your shoulders, your shoulders are over your hips, and your belly button is pulled up and under your ribs to engage the middle muscles and provide spinal support.

In This Chapter

- ◆ Arms in action
- ◆ Amazing legs and butt
- ◆ A total body fitness makeover
- ◆ Unleash your ab potential

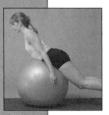
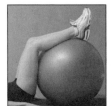
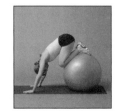
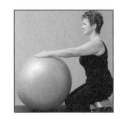
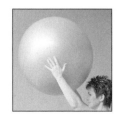
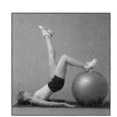

Chapter 5

The Body Ball Makeover

Now that you've developed the strength to hold your spine straight and strong, you'll tighten and tone those hard to hit areas such as your legs, hips, and arms. Combine the postural stability exercises that you've already done with these total body strength moves and you'll transform those villainous areas that seem to resist any muscle makeover.

Of course, it's your postural muscles that keep you afloat, only now you'll move your arms and legs to challenge them even more. But the pay off is huge: That solid muscle hiding behind a layer of fat will be revealed so that you now have shapely arms, leaner legs, and winning abs—the ideal body, if you like long and strong!

The Total Body Ball Makeover: Ball Intermediates

To round out your fitness formula, add some cardio to your week, increasing your time on the treadmill or stationary bike to 30–40 minutes. You can still do this chapter's total body workout after your cardio, if you feel up to it. By now, you should have enough strength and endurance to carry you through your day with plenty left over. If you have no plans to sweat-it-out beforehand, warm up with a five-minute walk or a light cardio workout.

The last chapter focused on developing postural strength, specifically spinal stability. You'll see those same exercises, only now you will train primary muscle groups with dumbbell weights. In other words, you'll engage your postural muscles while strength training your arms and legs.

Throughout your body, there are muscle groups that push and pull and often work together, co-contracting to help stabilize the joint attached. Your abdominals, for example, curl your spine forward while your back muscles arch it backwards. These opposite muscle actions (push and pull) support your delicate joints. When muscles are strong and balanced, then your joints are well protected and happy. And you'll look and feel good, too.

Defining every muscle in your body is virtually impossible, however, you'll have the opportunity to read about some primary muscles as you resistance train. More than likely, you've probably seen some of these exercises before but keep in mind, training on the ball makes them like new again!

The workout guidelines are as follows: You'll do two to three sets of 12–15 repetitions or reps of each exercise listed below. You may choose a 3, 5, or 8-pound dumbbell weight depending on your exercise history. Start light and then add more weight as you get stronger and more familiar with the ball. Reps are not the end goal, training with proper form is. Listen to your body.

If, for example, you can't keep your shoulders stable and find that they're creeping toward your ears, drop the weight. Poor alignment defeats the purpose of the exercise because you're strengthening the muscles to support poor alignment rather than good posture. Drop the weights if you feel fatigue or can't maintain a stable spine.

You're the boss of your body! With that, dust off your dumbbells, roll out your ball, and do this chapter's workout two to three times a week as part of a total body ball strength training program.

- Seated ball postural exercises: neutral and lateral rocks with hip circles for warm up. (see Chapter 4)
- Seated ball biceps curl
- Seated ball triceps extension
- Seated ball front raise
- Seated ball lateral raise
- Seated ball bent-Over fly
- Supine ball bridge with chest press
- Supine ball bridge with fly
- Spinal ball extension
- Spinal ball extension with legs lift
- One arm standing row with ball
- Abdominal ball curl
- Abdominal ball oblique curl
- Stationary ball plank
- Ball wall squat
- Ball plie wall squat
- Ball sideline outer thigh work
- Ball bridge with leg curl

Seated Ball Biceps Curl

Why it works: Sitting on the ball requires good posture. Now you'll train your trunk and tone the muscles of your upper arm: biceps and triceps. The biceps brachii define the front arm while triceps brachii define the back arm. Collectively, this group co-contracts to move your forearm. Of course, when toned, these muscles give you sexy and sleek arms plus strength to lift, lug, and carry all kinds of objects.

Start/Finish Position

1. Sit on the center of your ball with your knees hip-width apart, feet parallel, and firmly grounded to the floor. Maintain good alignment with a stable spine.

2. Hold a dumbbell in each hand and let your arms hang by your sides, palms up.

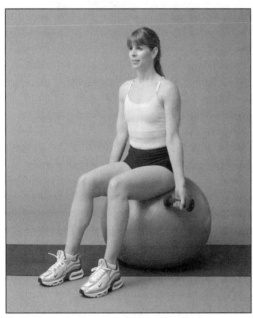

Biceps curl, start/finish.

Movement

3. In a count of four, lift your dumbbells slowly. Maintain a stable spine throughout the exercise!

4. In a count of four, lower your dumbbells.

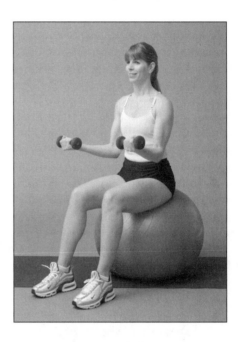

Biceps curl, movement.

Balancing Ball Tips

◆ When sitting on the ball, maintain a neutral spine as your arms work to challenge your trunk stability on the ball. Remember activate your deep stabilizing muscles by breathing, concentrating on your exhale to help keep you steady.

◆ When lifting your dumbbells, your pelvis may shift as well. Use your abdominals to keep you pelvis steady and you afloat.

◆ Keep your elbows stable, and anchored to your ribs.

Seated Ball Triceps Extension

Why it works: This exercise strengthens your triceps while engaging your middle muscles.

Start/Finish Position

1. Sit on the center of your ball with your knees hip-width apart, feet parallel, and firmly grounded to the floor. Maintain spinal alignment.

2. Hold a dumbbell in each hand.

3. Lift your arms over your head so your elbows bend forward as the weight drops behind your head, about a 90-degree angle.

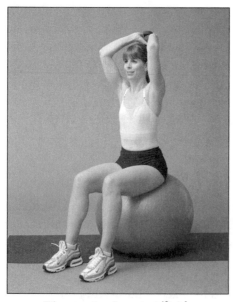

Triceps extension, start/finish.

Movement

4. In a count of four, lift your dumbbell to the ceiling. Your spine stability will be challenged as the weight lifts to the ceiling, so call on your middle muscles for support throughout this exercise.

5. In a count of four, lower your dumbbell to the starting position.

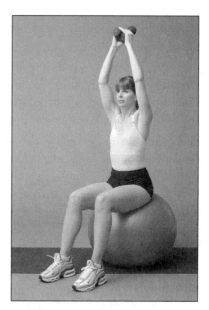

Triceps extension, movement.

Balancing Ball Tips

◆ When your arms are overhead, your trunk stability will be challenged, so activate your deep stabilizing muscles by breathing, concentrating on your exhale to help keep you steady.

◆ When lifting your dumbbells, your pelvis may shift as well. Maintain a stable pelvis at all times.

◆ Keep your elbows stable.

Seated Ball Front Raise

Why it works: Arm raises build shoulder strength plus sexier and shapelier shoulders. Without shoulder strength, you couldn't perform many day-to-day activities: lifting anything over your head, writing a simple note, playing sports, or strumming a musical instrument. These exercises strengthen your shoulder muscles or deltoids along with various upper back muscles. Start with lighter weights, because your shoulder joints are delicate and tend to be vulnerable to injury.

Start/Finish Position

1. Sit on the center of your ball with your knees hip-width apart, feet parallel and firmly grounded to the floor.
2. Inhale to roll your shoulders up to your ears, and then draw your shoulder blades down your back.
3. Pull your belly button up and in to support your spine. Maintain a stable spine.
4. Hold a dumbbell in each hand.
5. Let your arms hang by your sides, near the ball, so they are in line with your shoulders, palms down.

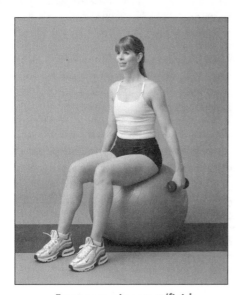

Front arm raise, start/finish.

Movement

6. In a count of four, lift your arms in front of you only to shoulder height. Don't lift your shoulders as your arms lift.
7. In a count of four, lower the weights.

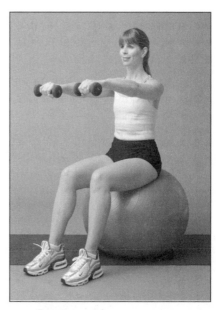

Front arm raise, movement.

Balancing Ball Tips

◆ Don't let your shoulders lift, as your arms do—stabilize your shoulder girdle by sliding your shoulder blades down your back.

◆ If you feel any neck strain, it's usually because the trapezius muscle is overcompensating for a weaker one. Use a lighter weight or don't train with dumbbells until you can work without strain.

◆ Don't lift your arms higher than your shoulders.

◆ Keep a soft bend in your elbows even though they're straight.

◆ Don't bend at the wrists.

Seated Ball Lateral Raise

Why it works: This exercise primarily strengthens the medial deltoid and challenges your trunk stability.

Start/Finish Position

1. Sit on the center of your ball with your knees hip-width apart, feet parallel, and firmly grounded to the floor.

2. Inhale to roll your shoulders up to your ears, and then draw your shoulder blades down your back.

3. Pull your belly button up and in to support your spine. Bend slightly forward from the waist, lifting your breastbone and maintaining a stable spine.

4. Hold a dumbbell in each hand.

5. Let your arms hang by your sides so they are in line with your shoulders, palms facing back.

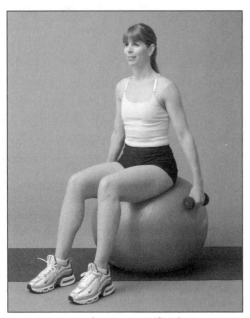

Lateral raise, start/finish.

Movement

6. In a count of four, lift your arms to your sides. Don't lift your shoulders as your arms lift.

7. In a count of four, lower the weights.

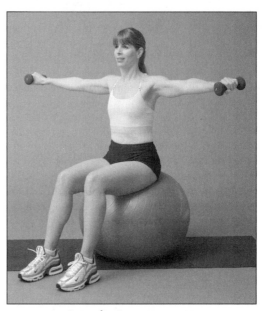

Lateral raise, movement.

Balancing Ball Tips

◆ Don't let your shoulders lift while your arms do.

◆ As you lean forward slightly, lift your breastbone and maintain a stable spine.

◆ Although you're leaning forward, pull your abdominal wall to your spine for trunk support.

◆ If you feel any neck strain, then usually it's your trapezius muscle compensating for a weaker muscle. Use a lighter weight or don't train with dumbbells until you can work without strain.

◆ Keep a soft bend in your elbows as you lift to the side.

◆ Don't bend at the wrists.

Seated Ball Bent-Over Fly

Why it works: This exercise primarily works the posterior deltoid while challenging your trunk.

Start/Finish Position

1. Sit on the center of your ball with your knees touching, feet parallel and firmly grounded to the floor.
2. Bend forward at the waist until your chest just about touches your thighs.
3. Lift your breastbone slightly to help maintain a stable spine.
4. Hold a dumbbell in each hand.
5. Let your arms dangle by your ankles, palms down, while gazing at the floor.

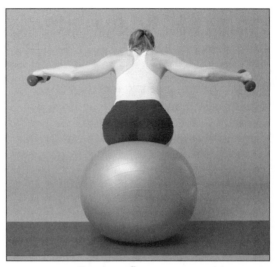

Bent-over fly, movement.

Balancing Ball Tips

◆ As you bend forward, don't round your back. Lift your breastbone to help align your spine and lift the pit of your belly to your spine.

◆ Contract your upper back muscles to lift your arms.

◆ Don't throw your arms into position. If you can't maintain smooth and controlled movements, use a lighter weight or don't use dumbbells at all.

◆ Because the posterior deltoid is usually a weak shoulder muscle, begin with a light weight.

◆ Imagine cracking a walnut between your shoulder blades to strengthen a variety of upper back muscles including your rhomboids, which are the muscles that sit between your shoulder blades to help pull them together.

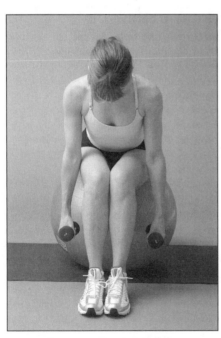

Bent-over fly, start/finish.

Movement

6. In a count of four, lift your arms up and out to the side, about shoulder height.
7. In a count of four, lower your arms. In both steps, imagine cracking a walnut between your shoulder blades.

On the Ball

If you need more of a ball challenge, move your feet closer together to decrease your base of stability.

Supine Ball Bridge with Chest Press

Why it works: These two exercises strengthen various muscle fibers of your chest: the pectoralis major and pectoralis minor. Collectively, these muscles assist in lifting your arms over your head, or when these muscles are tight, then they can restrict how high you can lift your arms over your head.

Start/Finish Position

1. Sit on the center of your ball.
2. Walk down ball into a supine ball bridge (see Chapter 4).
3. Hold a dumbbell in each hand.
4. Bend your elbows to your sides so they are in line with your shoulders, knuckles up.

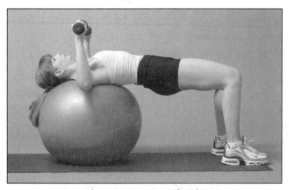

Chest press, start/finish.

Movement

5. In a count of four, press your arms to the ceiling.
6. In a count of four, lower your arms to the ball.

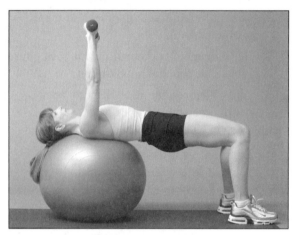

Chest press, movement.

Supine Ball Bridge with Fly

Why it works: This exercise works your chest muscles and tones your backside.

Start/Finish Position

1. Sit on the center of your ball.
2. Walk down the ball into a supine ball bridge (see Chapter 4).
3. Hold a dumbbell in each hand.
4. Lift your arms to the ceiling so your weights are even with your chest, palms in.

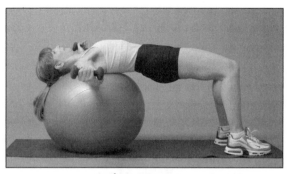

Fly, movement.

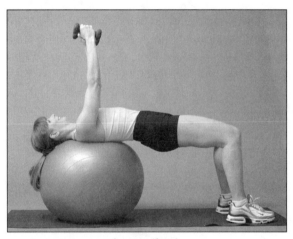

Fly start/finish.

Movement

5. In a count of four, open your arms to the side of your body.
6. Lower your arms so they're parallel to the floor, elbows slightly bent.
7. In a count of four, activate the muscles under your armpits to lift your arms to the ceiling.

Balancing Ball Tips

◆ Don't lower your hips. Try to remain in a Supine Ball Bridge position while your arms train the muscles in your chest.

◆ Your neck is in line with your spine and is supported by the ball.

◆ Engage your glutes to support your pelvis and hips and at the same time turn on your abdominals for trunk support, keeping the ball steady underneath you.

◆ Chest flys are long lever exercises so move slowly. Don't use momentum. Contract the muscles in your chest and activate the ones underneath your armpits to help create resistance for your muscles.

◆ Create resistance by slowly lowering your arms to increase the muscles' workload.

Spinal Ball Extension

Why it works: Sculpting your back is no longer a matter of back appeal, but back health. More people go to the doctor's office complaining of back pain than the common cold. Spinal extension strengthens your back muscles. Remember, spinal extension is tricky, so pay particular attention to how you move your body while extending your spine.

Start/Finish Position

1. Kneel in front of your ball, toes down.
2. Place your hips over the ball, so your legs are a little wider than your shoulders.
3. Drape torso over the ball.
4. Place your hands on the back of your thighs and gaze at the floor.

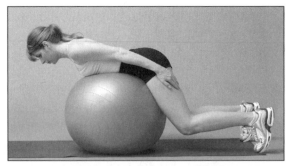

Spinal ball extension, start/finish.

Movement

5. Inhale to lift your chest off the ball; lengthen your spine.
6. Keep your head in line with your spine as your fingertips reach toward your heels.
7. Exhale to rest and drape over the ball.

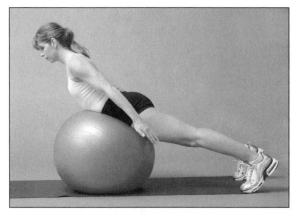

Spinal ball extension, movement.

Balancing Ball Tips

◆ Your neck is in line with your spine the whole time.

◆ Gaze at the floor.

◆ If you have a back injury, check with your doctor before doing extension.

Spinal Ball Extension with Leg Lift

Why it works: This exercise strengthens the muscles of your back while toning your buttocks and hamstrings.

Start/Finish Position

1. Kneel in front of your ball, toes down.
2. Drape over ball, placing your torso and hips on the ball.

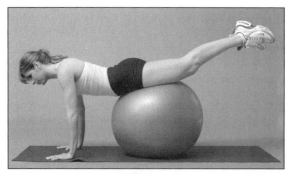

Legs lift, movement.

Balancing Ball Tips

◆ Before lifting your legs, focus on pulling the pit of your belly to your spine despite the ball supporting your abdomen. This action helps you balance as well.

◆ Keep your legs straight, lengthening through the heels to strengthen your hamstrings and glutes.

◆ Activate your glutes to lift your legs.

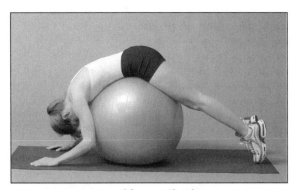

Legs lift, start/finish.

Movement

3. Walk your hands out so your pelvis is on the ball while gazing at the floor.
4. Lift your legs to the ceiling, activating your buttocks and hamstrings.
5. Hold this isometric contraction for five to eight counts.
6. Drape yourself over the ball to rest.

One Arm Standing Row with Ball

Why it works: This exercise strengthens your latissimus dorsi, which is a broad back muscle; it wraps from your back to your front ribs to provide trunk support in certain movements.

Start/Finish Position

1. Stand to the left of your ball.

2. Place your right hand on the apex of the ball.

3. Bend your knees, so they are at a 45-degree angle.

4. Pull your abdominals to your spine and lift your breastbone to keep your spine straight.

5. Hold a dumbbell weight in your left hand.

6. Straighten your arm to the floor, palms in, making sure your hand is in line with your shoulder.

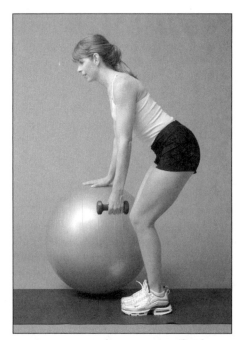

One arm standing row, start/finish.

Movement

7. In a count of four, bend your elbow and lift the back of your arm to the ceiling. The dumbbell weight glides past your rib cage as the elbow lifts high to ceiling. Keep your shoulders pulled away from your ears.

8. In a count of four, straighten your arm, controlling the weight as your hand lowers to the floor.

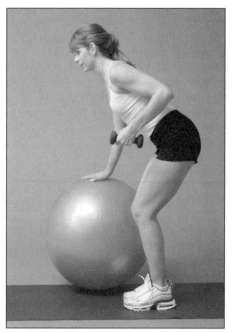

One arm standing row, movement.

Balancing Ball Tips

◆ Slide the weight past your ribs until your elbow lifts to the ceiling.

◆ Sit on your heels to get more leg work.

◆ If you want to advance this exercise, lift your leg to create a balance challenge.

Abdominal Ball Curl

Why it works: This exercise challenges and strengthens your abs while toning the backside of your body. Also, note that your upper back is off the ball, which will increase the workload for you abdominals.

Start/Finish Position

1. Sit on the center of your ball with your knees hip-width apart, feet parallel and firmly grounded to the floor.

2. Walk your feet away from the ball until your lower back presses against the ball. Your upper back, shoulders, and neck are off the ball.

3. Lace your fingers behind your head.

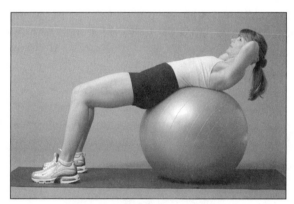

Abdominal ball curl, start/finish.

Movement

4. Inhale to prepare for the exercise.

5. Exhale to lift your shoulders up, about three inches off the ball and look to the wall in front of you.

6. Inhale to lower your body to the ball.

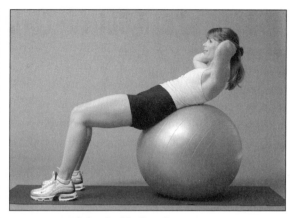

Abdominal ball curl, movement.

Balancing Ball Tips

◆ As you curl up, exhale and pull your ribs to your hips to engage your abs.

◆ Don't look at the ceiling; instead, gently guide your chin to your chest, maintaining length in the back of your neck.

◆ Exhale as much as you can while curling forward to engage your deep abdominals, specifically your transverse. Your goal is to create a tightening sensation around your waist as you exhale—your belly button drops to your spine.

◆ Don't jerk into position—exhale, curl, and control.

◆ Curl down with control, engaging all abdominal muscles.

◆ Keep the ball steady by using the muscles in your legs.

◆ Don't hold your breath.

◆ If you feel that these exercises are too easy, bring your feet closer together, decreasing your base of support.

◆ Don't pull on your head, which may cause neck strain.

Abdominal Ball Oblique Curl

Why it works: This abdominal exercise activates your oblique system.

Start/Finish Position

1. Sit on the center of your ball with your knees hip-width apart, feet parallel and firmly grounded to the floor.
2. Walk down the ball until your lower back is on the ball.
3. Lace your fingers behind your head.

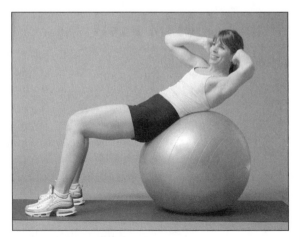

Abdominal ball oblique curl, movement.

Balancing Ball Tips

◆ As you curl up and twist, the rotation initiates from your rib cage. Your lower back must remain anchored to the ball.

◆ Focus on contracting your abdominals by first curling up and then using your elbow to twist a little higher.

◆ Don't hold your breath.

◆ Lace your fingertips loosely behind your head for support only. Don't pull on your head, which can create neck tension.

◆ If you need to increase the intensity, then bring your feet closer together.

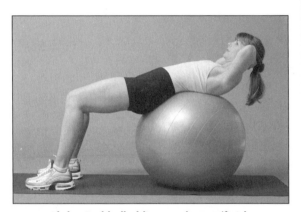

Abdominal ball oblique curl, start/finish.

Movement

4. Inhale to prepare for the movement.
5. Exhale to curl up and then turn your chest to the left so that your left elbow crosses your right thigh, ribs moving to your hips.
6. Inhale to lower your body to the ball.
7. Exhale to curl up and turn your chest to the right so that your right elbow crosses your left thigh, ribs moving to your hips.

Stationary Ball Plank

Why it works: This plank challenges and strengthens the muscles of your trunk, simultaneously. In fact, there is no better exercise for strengthening your core! This plank soars in intensity as you train with the ball farther from your trunk.

Start/Finish Position

1. Kneel in front of your ball.
2. Drape your abdomen and hips over the ball.
3. Place your hands on the floor in front of the ball.

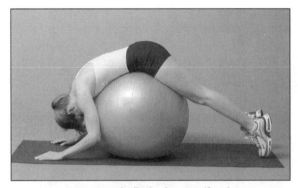

Stationary ball plank, start/finish.

Movement

4. Walk your hands away from the ball so it rolls near your knees with your legs straight.
5. Lift your belly button to the ceiling to help support your trunk and hold this plank for 10–15 breaths, pulling your navel to your spine on each exhale.
6. Drape over the ball to stretch your lower back.

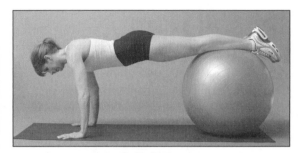

Stationary ball plank, movement.

Balancing Ball Tips

◆ If you have a shoulder, neck, or back injury, please check with your doctor before doing this exercise.

◆ Hug your abs to your spine the whole time to lessen the strain on your lower back.

◆ Holding this plank takes lots of upper body strength so pay attention to your shoulder alignment: Wrists are directly under your shoulders. To help keep your shoulders in place, draw your shoulder blades down your back.

◆ Don't let your shoulders elevate toward your ears.

◆ If you have any lower back pain, check your alignment. Are you lifting your navel to your spine, keeping your midsection stable? Check your hand placement. If your hands are too far from the ball, then walk them back towards the ball to lessen the strain on your trunk. If the pain persists, then stop this exercise.

◆ Remember, your goal is to begin by aligning your body correctly only then can your muscles strengthen to support good form.

Ball Wall Squat

Why it works: Squats develop long and sexy legs by strengthening just about every leg muscles at the same time: abductors, adductors, hamstrings, and quadriceps. Strong legs are not only sexy, but they're functional—they keep you moving and can protect you from injury. Squats in general work your leg muscles synergistically for a balanced lower body, but mainly target the front thigh muscles or *quadriceps.*

Body Ball Language

Collectively, your quadriceps or quads make up four muscles of the front or your thigh. They originate on your thigh bone or femur and run in various directions past your knee: the rectus femoris is the big muscle of the front thigh, vastus medialis attaches to the inner front portion of the femur, the vastus lateralis attaches to the outer front, and the vastus intermedius attaches between the two.

1. Stand with your fitness ball between your mid-back and a wall, with your feet a little wider than hip-width apart.
2. Align your knees so they track between your second and third toes.
3. Lift your breastbone to straighten your spine.
4. Place hands on your thighs for support.

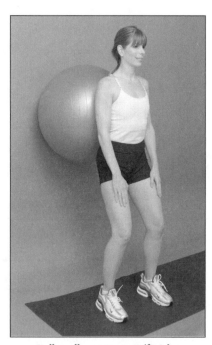

Ball wall squat, start/finish.

Movement

5. In a count of four, lower your bottom to the floor so your thighs are parallel with the ground.
6. Place the majority of your body weight in your heels to prevent your knees from extending past your toes.
7. In a count of four, straighten your legs.
8. Lift your belly button to your spine for trunk support and to help keep the ball steady.

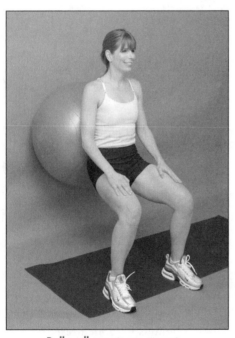

Ball wall squat, movement.

Balancing Ball Tips

◆ If you feel any strain in your knees, check your alignment. Align your knees so they track between your second and third toes. If you still feel any strain, try sitting back on your heels.

◆ Lift your breastbone to help keep your spine stable and straight. Don't lean forward.

◆ Lift from the top of your head to keep your spine active and straight.

◆ If you need more of a challenge, raise your arms so that they're parallel to the floor.

Ball Plié Wall Squat

Why it works: Ball Plié wall squats also strengthen your leg muscles but specifically target inner thighs. Your inner thighs muscles, or adductors, are long and slender and tend to be hard to tone. However, when they are toned, these muscles accentuate your legs (most beautifully) plus assist in moving your legs across the midline of your body to help stabilize your pelvis so you can walk, run, climb, and lunge.

Start/Finish Position

1. Stand with your fitness ball between your mid-back and a wall.

2. Open your legs twice hip-width apart and turn your toes out.

3. Align your knees over your second and third toes.

4. Lift your breastbone to keep your spine straight and stable.

5. Lower your arms between your thighs.

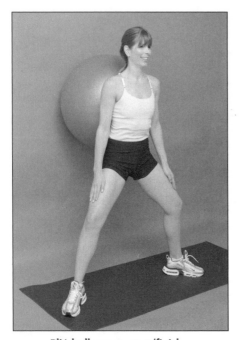

Plié ball squat, start/finish.

Movement

6. In four counts, lower bottom to the floor so your thighs are parallel with the ground, if you can. Your knees should not extend past your toes.

7. In a count of four, straighten your legs as you engage the muscles between your legs.

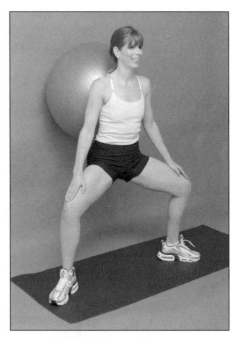

Plié ball squat, movement.

Balancing Ball Tips

◆ You can use a dumbbell weight such as 10–25 pounds for added resistance. Hold the head of a dumbbell with both hands and let it dangle between your thighs.

◆ Imagine squeezing a ball between your legs to get the maximum inner thigh and butt activation.

◆ Stand tall and lift your chest.

Ball Sideline Outer Thigh Work

Why it works: This exercise strengthens and tones your outer thighs (the abductors) and test your balance and coordination while you're in a side position on the ball. These muscles move your legs away from your body. They, unfortunately, tend to tap the fat in the form of dimples. Your adductors and abductors co-contract to stabilize your leg as you balance and as you move—like when you walk, run, or lunge.

Start/Finish Position

1. Lie on your side over the ball.
2. Bend your bottom leg to help stabilize you.
3. Lower your top leg to the floor.
4. Align your head with your spine.
5. If you feel very wobbly, then remain in this position until you can control the ball underneath you.

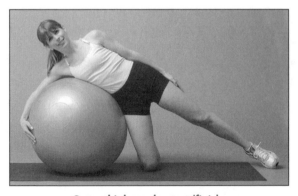

Outer thigh work, start/finish.

Movement

6. In a count of four, lift your leg up to the ceiling.
7. In a count of four, lower your leg to the floor.

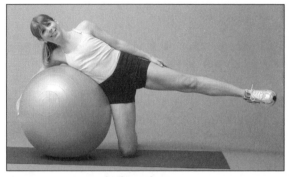

Outer thigh work, movement.

Balancing Ball Tips

◆ If you feel very wobbly, place the ball against the wall.
◆ Keep your knee turned to the side to work the outer thigh to its fullest.

Ball Bridge with Leg Curl

Why it works: Leg curls lift your derriere and tone the muscles of your backside, which include your *gluteus maximus* and back thigh muscles, *hamstrings*. Meanwhile, you're still training the muscles that provide pelvic and trunk stability.

Start/Finish Position

1. Lie on your back with the ball under your knees so it rest against the back of your thighs—knees bent in a 90-degree position.
2. Lengthen your arms by your sides, palms down.

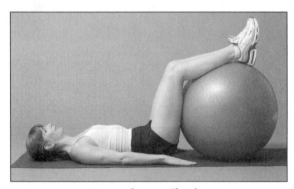

Leg curls, start/finish.

Movement One

3. Walk the ball out so it's under your calves.
4. Lift your hips to the ceiling so your back is off the floor.
5. Secure your heels in the center of your ball.

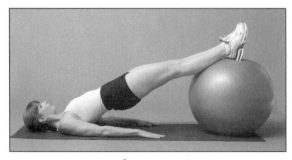

Leg curls, movement one.

Movement Two

6. In a count of four, bend your knees and use the heels of your feet to roll the ball toward your butt—in one motion.
7. In a count of four, roll the ball away from your bottom while maintaining the lift your bottom.

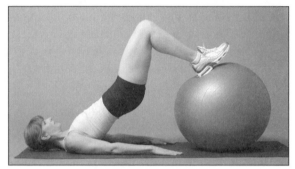

Leg curls, movement two.

Balancing Ball Tips

◆ Your shoulders, pelvis, and knees are in one line.
◆ Don't forget to pull your belly button to your spine, creating a strong core.
◆ Remember, this gravity-defying butt move must initiate from your glutes and hamstrings.
◆ Press the palms of your hands into the floor to help stabilize your trunk while your legs move the ball.
◆ If you feel that your pelvis is not stable, don't move the ball. You must stay lifted in your bottom and even in your hip bones to strengthen the muscles correctly.

Body Ball Language

Ball exercises such as supine ball bridge and bridge on the floor tighten and tone the backside of your body. The biggest and most stubborn muscle is your butt muscle, the **gluteus maximus** while your **hamstrings** are comprised of three muscles making up your back thighs: biceps femoris, semitendinosus, and semimembranosus.

Congratulations

Congratulations again! With a lot of hard work you should see visible results along with some definite definition in your body. Remember, this workout trains primary muscles, and with any luck you're on your way to a body makeover.

The Least You Need to Know

◆ These exercises strengthen your postural muscles while sculpting your arms and legs.

◆ Throughout your body, muscles or muscle groups have opposite actions and often work together to co-contract to help stabilize the attached joint.

◆ If you need more of a ball challenge, move your feet closer together to decrease your base of stability.

◆ Reps are not the end goal; training with good alignment is.

In This Chapter

- ◆ Get lean all over
- ◆ Manipulate your metabolism
- ◆ Strike a pose between balance and strength
- ◆ Multi-muscle training is a time-saver

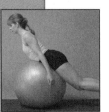 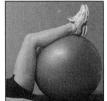 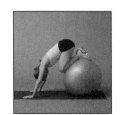 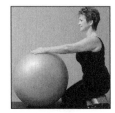 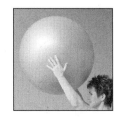 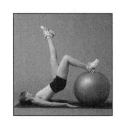

Chapter 6

Mind-Body Ball Blitz

You multitask all day long, now you'll multitask your muscles! The truth is, your muscles love working in groups, and it's an effective way to manipulate your resting metabolism (the number of calories your body uses when doing nothing). That's why this va-va-voom workout blends balance challenges and strength moves. So you burn calories and strengthen your muscles *and* your mind.

Speaking of burn, multi-muscle training ignites your internal power and forces your body into action. Balance requires muscles! Muscles burn fat! Interested yet?

Mind–Body Ball Blitz: Advanced

To get a complete workout, do some steady-state training at an easy-to-moderate pace for 50–60 minutes to help burn maximum calories at least four to five days a week—remember you want to change your body! If you can carry on a conversation during your cardio, you're keeping a moderate pace. When you exercise at a lower intensity, you're able to keep going, which means your metabolism keeps at it longer as well. Choose your cardio—enjoy a walk with your dogs, exercise on the elliptical trainer, or step your heart out—just shoot for 60 minutes. By now, you should have plenty of strength and some endurance, so you can either do this total body ball workout after your cardio or on an alternate day depending on your fitness plan.

With your new strength, you'll now strike a pose! In other words, you will improve your balance and coordination skills by reducing the number of points you balance on. If, for example, an exercise called for standing on both legs, you'll now stand on one.

The workout guidelines are as follows: You'll do two to three sets of 12–15 repetitions or reps of each exercise listed below. You may still choose a 3, 5, or 8-pound dumbbell weights but try to lift heavier than the last workout. If you feel fatigue or can't balance with good form, drop down in weight or don't use them at all. Do this workout two to three times a week as part of a total body ball strength training program.

- Seated postural ball exercises: neutral, lateral rocks with hip circles (see Chapter 4)
- Ball wall squat with biceps curls
- Ball plié wall squat with upright row
- Ball single leg lunge
- One arm standing row with single leg ball squat

Ball Blowout

Balance recruits many of the body's deep stabilizing muscles. Most are underused, and therefore weak, which can result in an injury.

- Stationary ball plank
- Stationary ball plank with leg extension
- Stationary ball pike
- Stationary ball push-up
- Spinal ball extension
- Spinal ball extension with triceps kickback
- Ball bridge with leg curls and leg extension
- Inner thigh squeeze with abdominal ball curl
- Reverse ball curl
- Scissor ball rotation

On the Ball

Balance requires a joint effort from multiple muscles. Two in particular are adductors and abductors, which co-contract to keep you standing on one leg. When strong, these two muscles co-contract to help you balance in every step you take.

Ball Wall Squat with Biceps Curl

Why it works: This exercise combines arm and legs movement to test your coordination and strengthen your quadriceps and biceps.

Start/Finish Position

1. Stand with your fitness ball between your mid-back and a wall; feet are a little wider than hip-length.
2. Align your knees between your second and third toes.
3. Hold a dumbbell in each hand.
4. Let your arms hang by your sides, palms up.

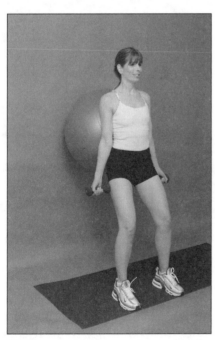

Wall squat with biceps curl, start/finish.

Movement

5. In a count of four, lower your bottom toward the floor so your thighs are parallel with the ground and do a biceps curl—at the same time! (See Chapter 5.)

6. In a count of four, straighten your legs and arms, contracting your abs to help stabilize the ball.

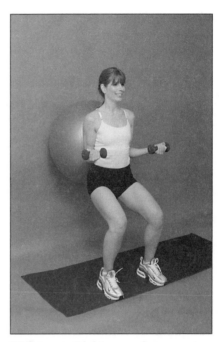

Wall squat with biceps curl, movement.

Balancing Ball Tips

◆ This exercise is meant to coordinate the movement of your arms and legs, testing your balance and coordination. If you feel uncomfortable with the movement, work the squat first, and then do a set of biceps curls.

◆ Your knees should not extend past your toes. Place your body weight in your heels. If you feel knee strain, make sure that your knees track between the second and third toes.

◆ Stand tall—lift your breastbone to keep your spine straight.

◆ Lift the top of your head to the ceiling to keep your spine active and straight.

◆ Exhale deeply to create support for your spine, strengthen your abdominals, and to help steady the ball.

Ball Plié Wall Squat with Upright Row

Why it works: This exercise strengthens your inner thighs, buttocks, mid-deltoids, and upper back muscles.

Start/Finish Position

1. Stand with your fitness ball between your mid-back and a wall.

2. Open your legs twice hip-width apart and turn your toes out.

3. Align your knees between your second and third toes.

4. Lift your breastbone to help straighten your spine.

5. Hold a dumbbell in each hand, letting your arms hang between your thighs, palms in.

7. Turn your elbows out to your sides, bringing the dumbbell heads together.

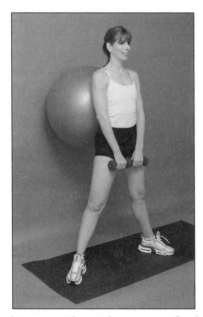

Plié squat with upright row, start/finish.

Movement

8. In a count of four, lower your bottom to the floor and lift your dumbbells to your chest at the same time. Your thighs move parallel with the floor.

9. In a count of four, straighten your legs and lower your arms toward the floor.

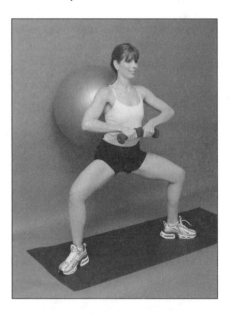

Plié squat with upright row, movement.

Balancing Ball Tips

◆ As you lift your dumbbells into an upright row, press your shoulder blades down your back so your shoulders don't elevate as your arms lift.

◆ Maintain a neutral wrist position.

◆ Imagine squeezing a ball between your legs to feel the contraction in the deepest inner thigh and meaty portions of your butt.

◆ Stand tall, lifting your chest and pulling your shoulders back.

◆ For extra support, use your breath to help stabilize your body, inhale on the way down, and exhale on the way up to engage your abs and help stabilize the ball behind your back.

Ball Single Leg Lunge

Why it works: This exercise blends butt and balance work while strengthening just about every muscle in the stationary leg, which include delicate muscles in the foot, ankle, knee, and hip.

Start/Finish Position

1. Stand in front of your fitness ball with your feet hip-width apart.

2. Place the top of your right foot on the ball so your knee faces the floor.

3. Let your hands drop to your sides, fingertips lengthening to the floor.

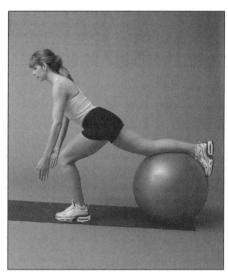

Single leg lunge, movement.

Balancing Ball Tips

◆ Don't lean over while lunging; rather, lift your breastbone to help lengthen and lift your spine.

◆ If you feel very unstable, place your fingertips on the wall for support. To get in the best position, measure an arm's length from the wall and stand there.

◆ The knee of your standing leg is directly over your heel.

◆ Point your hip bones toward the floor, keeping them as even as possible, especially as the leg moving the ball rolls it back.

◆ Sink down into your thighs as you lunge to activate more leg muscles.

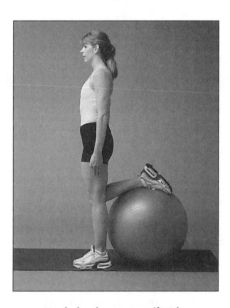

Single leg lunge start/finish.

Movement

4. In a count of four, bend the standing leg and roll the ball behind you, guiding it with your foot.

5. Lower yourself until the standing leg is in a deep lunge with the thigh almost parallel to the floor.

6. Lift your breastbone to lengthen and lift your spine—remember neutral and stable.

7. In a count of four, slowly straighten your leg.

On the Ball

Standing on one leg builds strength in the many muscles of the foot, ankle, knee, and thigh, which can increase your balance skills and protect you from injury.

One Arm Standing Row with Single Leg Ball Squat

Why it works: This exercise strengthens your lats while challenging your balance. Strong lats, in addition to strong glutes, can help support your pelvis as well as increase your balance skills, making this an ideal exercise.

Start/Finish Position

1. Stand to the left of your ball.
2. Place your right hand on the apex of the ball.
3. Bend your knees, so they are at a 45-degree angle.
4. Pull your abdominals to your spine and lift your breastbone to keep your spine straight.
5. Hold a dumbbell weight in your left hand and straighten your arm to the floor, palm in making sure your hand is in line with your shoulder.
6. Lift your left leg so that it's parallel to the floor and straighten your right leg—it's okay if your right knee is slightly bent.

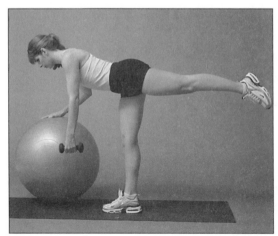

One arm standing row with one leg ball wall squat, start/finish.

Movement

7. In a count of four, bend your elbow and lift the back of your arm to the ceiling. The dumbbell weight glides past your rib cage as the elbow lifts high to ceiling.
8. Keep your shoulders pulled away from your ears.
9. In a count of four, straighten your arm, controlling the weight as your hand lowers to the floor.

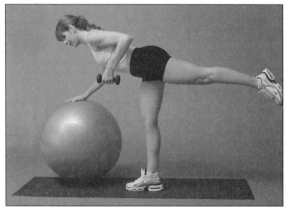

One arm standing row with one leg ball wall squat, movement.

Balancing Ball Tips

◆ Slide the weight past your ribs until your elbow lifts to the ceiling.
◆ Lift the pit of your belly to the ceiling to help support your trunk and keep you steady.
◆ Don't lift your leg high if you can't control the ball.
◆ Focus—it's much more difficult than it looks.
◆ After completing 8–12 reps, repeat with opposite leg and arm.

Stationary Ball Plank

Why it works: Planks strengthen many muscles at the same time, challenge your core; tone your arms and shoulders; and tighten your butt, hips, and legs. It's the ultimate multi-muscle move, especially this plank, which is the most difficult of all the planks you've done up to this point. The ball rolls toward your shins or ankles; therefore, gravity can push down on a bigger base, creating a big challenge!

Start/Finish Position

1. Kneel in front of your ball.
2. Drape your abdomen and hips over the ball.
3. Place your hands on the floor in front of the ball.

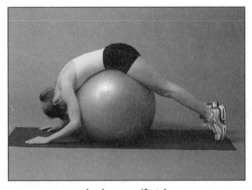

Plank, start/finish.

Movement One

4. Walk your hands out until the ball rolls toward your shins. Your body is absolutely straight, contract between your thighs for extra inner thigh support.
5. Lift your belly button to the sky.
6. Drape your body over the ball for a lower back stretch.

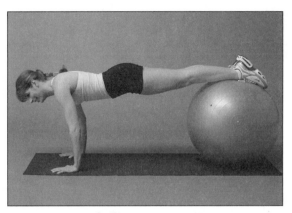

Plank, movement one.

Balancing Ball Tips

◆ If you have a shoulder or neck injury, leave this exercise out.

◆ To alleviate wrist pressure, consider using a pair of dumbbell weights to help keep your wrists in a neutral position.

◆ Hand placement is an absolute must. You must have your wrists directly under your shoulders and your shoulder blades sliding down your back to create shoulder stability.

◆ If you feel pressure in your lower back, pull your belly button to your spine with every deep exhale.

◆ If the ball wobbles, try exhaling deeper and contracting between your thighs to steady it.

Stationary Ball Plank with Leg Extension

Why it works: Balance and coordination aren't ignored in this plank, which requires plenty of both—and then some major strength. This plank engages and strengthens just about every muscle in your body, but targets your hamstrings and butt.

Movement Two

7. Engage the muscles between your thighs for extra support.
8. Lift the pit of your belly to your spine.
9. When ready, lift your left leg and hold this contraction for three to five breaths.
10. Lower your leg.
11. Repeat leg extension on the opposite leg.
12. Drape over the ball to stretch your lower back.

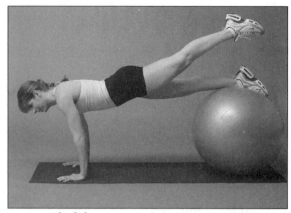

Plank leg extensions, movement two.

On the Ball

Find your focus! Learning to balance on the ball can also improve your levels of concentration.

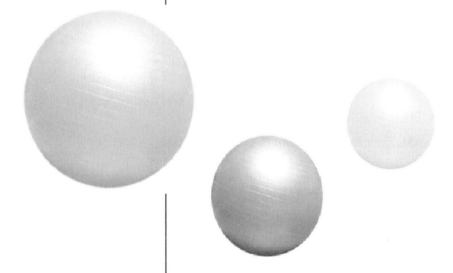

Stationary Ball Pike

Why it works: This extreme plank is the ultimate body and balance challenge. Pike activates just about every muscle in your body including your mind and propels your core into action. Find your focus!

Start/Finish Position

1. Kneel in front of your ball.
2. Drape your abdomen and hips over the ball.
3. Place your hands on the floor in front of the ball.
4. Crawl on top of the ball until your knees are tucked underneath you, shins resting on top of the ball, which is a nice stretch!

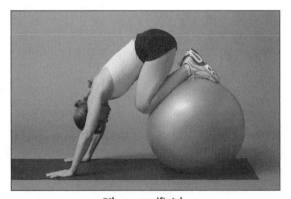

Pike, start/finish.

Movement

5. Align your wrists directly under your shoulders, with elbows secure, but not locked.
6. Inhale to find your focus.
7. Exhale to lift your hips to the sky, forcing your abs into action.

8. Hold this pike for five to eight breaths, exhaling deeply to perfect your form—hips over your shoulders and shoulders over your wrists so your torso is in a straight line.
9. Relax by tucking your knees underneath you on the ball.

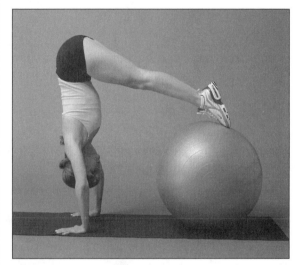

Pike, movement.

Balancing Ball Tips

◆ The length of your trunk, from your wrists to your hips, makes a straight line.

◆ Find your focus by gazing at the ball.

◆ Continue to breathe deeply to hold the pike with good form—and engage your abs to the max.

◆ Don't look at the floor. Gaze at the ball to lengthen your neck.

Stationary Ball Push-Up

Why it works: This Plank works all the same muscles and targets your shoulder and chest muscles.

Start/Finish Position

1. Kneel in front of your ball.
2. Drape your abdomen and hips over the ball.
3. Place your hands on the floor in front of the ball.
4. Walk your hands out until the ball rolls toward your shins. Open your hands so they're slightly wider than your shoulders.
5. Point your fingertips in, slightly.
6. With your body absolutely straight, contract between your thighs for extra inner thigh support.
7. Lift your belly button to the sky.

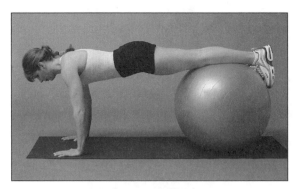

Push-up, start/finish.

Movement

8. In a count of four, maintain your plank as you bend your elbows, lowering your nose to the floor.
9. In a count of four, push up so your body is in a plank position.

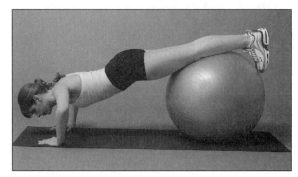

Push-up, movement.

Balancing Ball Tips

◆ Contract your abdominals.
◆ Remember, head to heel like steel—meaning your entire body is active and straight even as you lower yourself toward the floor.
◆ Align your wrists under your elbows with elbows parallel to each other.

Spinal Ball Extension

Why it works: As you now know, extension is vital in the development of a healthy spine. Remember, your spinal extensors co-contract with the abdominals to create a strong core; therefore, spinal extension can strengthen your back while stretching your abdominals. But that's not all. Extension on the ball strengthens your back muscles and targets the muscles in your legs as they engage to stabilize you.

Start/Finish Position

1. Kneel in front of your ball, toes down.
2. Place your hips over the ball so that your legs are hip-width apart.
3. Drape over the ball.
4. Lace your fingers and place your hands behind your head.
5. Gaze at the floor.

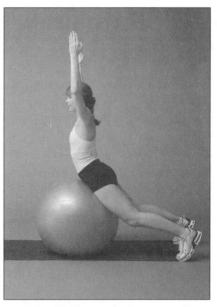

Spinal ball extension, movement.

Balancing Ball Tips

◆ Elongate slowly through each bone of your spine. Remember, move slowly and thoughtfully as you strengthen your back.

◆ Lift the top of your head toward the ceiling to lengthen your spine.

◆ Slide the shoulder blades down your back to stabilize your upper back.

◆ Keep your head in line with spine the whole time.

◆ Keep your abs active while your legs and arms work to stabilize you.

◆ If you're wobbly or feel strain in your lower back, widen your legs to about shoulder-width apart.

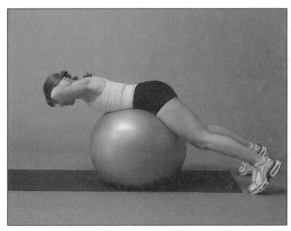

Spinal ball extension, start/finish.

Movement

6. Inhale to lift your chest off the ball, straightening your spine from the top of your head.
7. Reach your fingertips to the ceiling.
8. Complete three to five breaths.
9. Drape over ball.

On the Ball

As you multitask your muscles, you're multitasking your joints. Work cautiously so as not to put any undo strain on your joints. There's an added benefit to multi-muscle training; it's a time-saver.

Spinal Ball Extension with Triceps Kickback

Why it works: This extension strengthens your back muscles while toning your triceps.

Start/Finish Position

1. Kneel in front of your ball, toes down.
2. Place your hips over the ball, so your legs are about shoulder-width apart.
3. Hold a dumbbell weight in each hand.
4. Place your hands on the ball so the weights are by your sides. Your elbows are near your ribs and lifted to the ceiling, palms in.
5. Gaze at the floor.

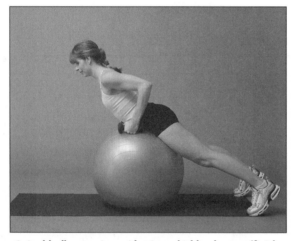

Spinal ball extension with triceps kickback, start/finish.

Movement

6. In a count of four, straighten your arms behind you, pressing the dumbbells' heads toward the ceiling.
7. In a count of four, bend your elbows and lower the dumbbells to the ball.

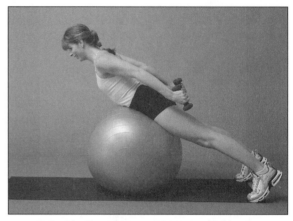

Spinal ball extension with triceps kickback, movement.

Balancing Ball Tips

◆ Try to maintain an extension of the spine while training your triceps.

◆ Keep your elbows near your ribs and lifted high to the ceiling.

◆ Relax your neck, and gaze at the floor.

◆ Don't swing the movement. Slow and controlled moves are better for your body and gentler to your delicate joints.

Ball Bridge with Leg Curls and Leg Extensions

Why it works: These advanced leg curls define your bottom and hamstrings, challenge your pelvic stability, strengthen your core, and improve your balance and coordination.

Start/Finish Position

1. Lie on your back with the ball under your knees and against the back of your thighs so that your knees are bent in a 90-degree position.
2. Lengthen your arms by your sides, palms down.

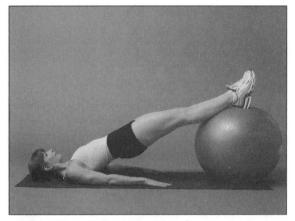

Ball bridge with leg extension curls, movement one.

Movement Two

5. Lift your right leg off the ball, reaching your toes to the ceiling.

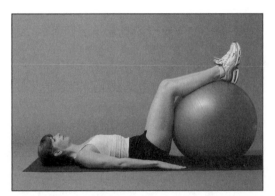

Ball bridge with leg extension curls, start/finish.

Movement One

3. Walk the ball out so that it's under your calves. Lift your hips to the sky so your back is off the floor.
4. Plant your heels into the center of your ball.

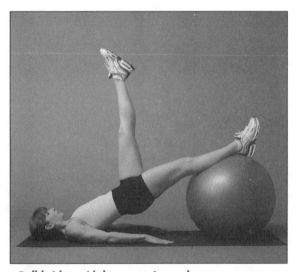

Ball bridge with leg extension curls, movement two.

Movement Three

6. In one motion, bend your right knee and use the heel of your right foot to roll the ball toward your butt while lifting your bottom.

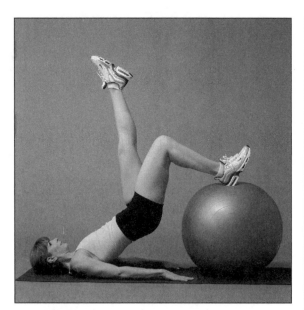

Ball bridge with leg extension curls, movement three.

Balancing Ball Tips

- Focus on keeping your hips even and your pelvis stable as you lift your leg. The tendency is for your hip to droop.
- Align your shoulders and pelvis so they form one line.
- Activate your core by dropping your belly button to your spine.
- You might feel a slight burn in the working hamstring. You don't have to roll the ball in as much.
- Press the palms of your hands into the floor to help lift and stabilize your torso as your legs work.

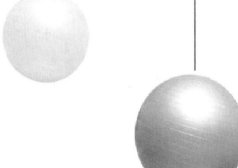
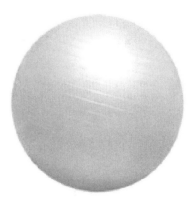

Inner Thigh Ball Squeeze with Abdominal Curl

Why it works: This ab exercise challenges your abdominals and tones and strengthens your inner thighs.

Start/Finish Position

1. Lie on your back with your legs extended, flex your feet.
2. Place the ball between your shins, squeezing the ball.
3. Lengthen your arms by your sides, palms down.

Movement

4. Inhale to curl your chin to your chest and lift your upper back off the floor; gaze between your thighs.
5. Stay lifted as you exhale dropping the pit of your belly to the floor, squeezing the air out.
6. Inhale to lower your back to the floor.

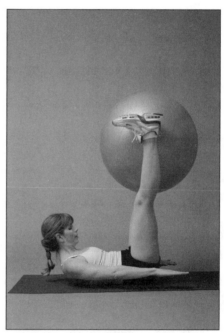

Inner thigh ball squeeze with abdominal curl, movement.

Balancing Ball Tips

◆ Gaze between your thighs.
◆ Press the palm of your hands into the floor for support, if needed.
◆ If you feel any strain in your neck, don't lift your head off the floor.
◆ This inner thigh abdominal curl is easier than the reverse curl, which is the next exercise. You can stop after this exercise or if you want more abdominal challenge then attempt the reverse curl.

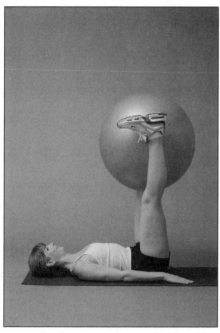

Inner thigh ball squeeze with abdominal curl, start/finish.

Reverse Ball Curl

Why it works: This exercise works the abdominals and inner thighs while challenging your stable pelvis.

Start/Finish Position

1. Lie on your back with your knees bent.
2. Place the ball between your shins, squeezing the ball.
3. Lace your fingers and place them behind your head.

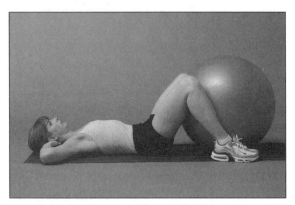

Reverse curl, start/finish.

Movement One

4. Inhale to curl your chin to your chest and lift your upper back off the floor, gazing between your thighs.

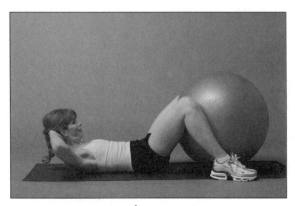

Reverse curl, movement one.

Movement Two

5. Stay lifted as you exhale to move your knees toward your chest, squeezing the air out.
6. Inhale to lower your feet to the floor.

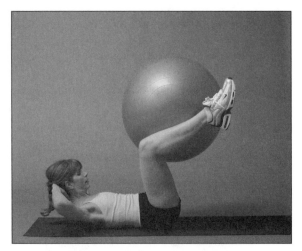

Reverse curl, movement two.

Balancing Ball Tips

- Make sure your pelvis remains in a neutral spine the whole time.
- As your legs return to the floor their weight may pull your lower back into an arch, focus on dropping your belly button to your spine, which also helps stabilize your pelvis.
- Keep your torso stable as the movement of your legs challenge and strengthen your abdominals.
- Don't look up at the ceiling. Instead, look between your thighs.
- If you can't maintain a stable pelvis, you don't have to lower your feet to the floor. Take them to the point in which you feel challenged yet stable.

Scissor Ball Rotation

Why it works: This advanced exercise works the muscles of your waist and your inner thighs, too.

Start/Finish Position

1. Lie on your back, place the ball between your shins, and squeeze it to strengthen your inner thighs.

3. Lengthen your arms out to the side, so they make a "T" with your body, with your palms down.

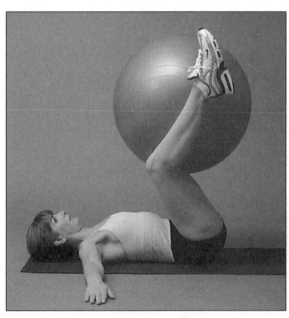

Scissor rotation, start/finish.

Movement

4. Inhale to prepare for the movement.

5. Exhale to rotate your legs to the right as far as you can without lifting your shoulders off the floor.

6. Inhale while moving your legs to center.

7. Exhale to rotate your legs to the left as far as you can without lifting your shoulders off the floor.

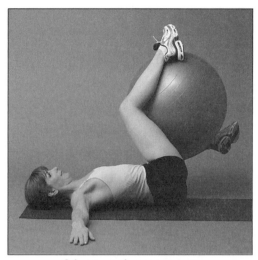

Scissor rotation, movement.

Balancing Ball Tips

◆ If you have a lower back injury, leave this exercise out.

◆ Press the palms of your hands into the floor to help support your torso.

◆ If your chin juts to the ceiling, creating a severe arch in your neck, place a small towel behind your head to lift your head off the floor.

Okay, now you're really done. You should feel really good about your body. Of course, if you want more ball challenges, turn to Pilates on the ball.

The Least You Need to Know

◆ There's nothing like the ball to boost your metabolism and get your best body.

◆ This total body workout moves multiple muscles while blending balance challenges and strength moves.

◆ Multi-muscle training calls for plenty of core strength, which is your body's source of power (internal power).

◆ Balance requires muscles and muscles burn fat, which is why multi-muscle training revs up your metabolism.

◆ Multi-muscle training is a time-saver in the gym.

In This Part

7 The Poised Pilates Ball Body

8 The Mind-Bending Ball Workout

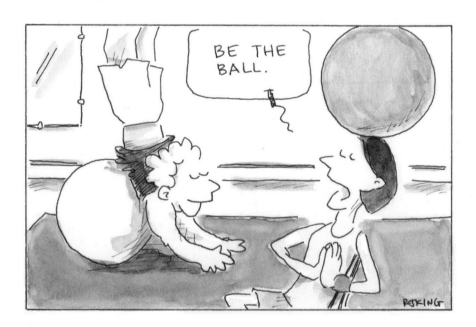

Part 3

It's a Mind–Body Ball Thing

Here's a side of the mat you might know about: Pilates on the ball! Here I provide general information about Pilates and why the ball and Pilates make an awesome twosome. Chapter 7 transforms the most stubborn of poochy abs by training your postural muscles. Chapter 8 is Pilates on the ball.

In This Chapter

- ◆ Defining Pilates
- ◆ The beginning: Joseph Pilates
- ◆ Six guiding principles
- ◆ Ball makes Pilates sense

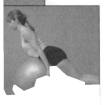
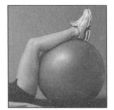
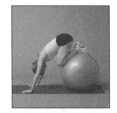
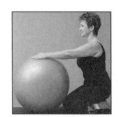
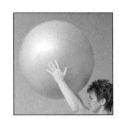
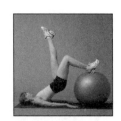

Chapter 7

The Poised Pilates Ball Body

Imagine for a minute having a deep sense of strength penetrating your midsection. Of course, this strength contours your waist so that you can see your curves. It's not the superficial six-pack-ab kind of strength that you see in fitness magazines, but a deep strength that gives you enough energy to keep you going when you think you can't go on.

Yet the most popular ab exercise around, the stomach crunch, can't do this. But then again, you probably already know this: You've set your own crunch-a-thon record.

So, here's some good fitness news. A stomach crunch is no longer the golden standard of abdominal exercises. But before you roll up your mat, you should know that fit, fabulous abs go beyond good looks. Fitness experts now know that a strong core is your body's source of power and is vital to keeping you healthy. Enter Pilates.

Defining Pilates?

Pilates is a smarter strategy to amazing abs, long and lean legs, and a lengthened body with perfect posture. Pilates, pronounced "puh-LAH-teez," is a total mind and body workout invented by Joseph Pilates (1880–1967). You can sculpt and shape your body without bulking up your muscles. Since every Pilates exercise aligns the spine and focuses on postural harmony, Pilates taps into your body's source of strength—your core!

On the Ball

With Pilates, you're stabilizing and strengthening your postural muscles in a variety of ways, which is why the ball blends with Pilates.

The Beginning: Joseph Pilates

Joseph Pilates used a variety of disciplines, from Eastern and Western philosophies, to invent a hybrid exercise method of conditioning. He was driven by his own sickly childhood. To overcome his serious health conditions such as asthma and rheumatic fever, he devoted his life to studying modalities to strengthen his body. Perhaps instinctively, he knew that the body would re-harmonize and heal itself given the opportunity. So, he began an intensive study of a variety of fitness regimes and modalities, from east to west. And in the end, became an accomplished athlete mastering a variety of sports such as gymnastics, boxing, and body building—just to name a few.

Joseph Pilates found great value in Eastern traditions such as yoga but also enjoyed the physicality of Western approaches to physical fitness. Pilates combines both.

During the First World War, Joseph Pilates was imprisoned as a German national in England. While captive, he taught his exercises (which make up the traditional mat work today) to other internees and continued to experiment with new exercises. He attached springs to hospital beds, for example, so that inactive casualties of war could exercise. This idea became the prototype for a piece of equipment called the Cadillac, which is used today in many Pilates studios.

His methods caught the attention of many, from the elite British military to prominent athletes. He continued training after returning home to Germany. As his vision of the ideal fitness regime gained in popularity, the new German army became interested in Mr. Pilates' methods and wanted him to train them. But he declined the offer and soon left for America.

On the Ball

"Movements are planned to relieve the heart, lungs, and liver of constriction caused by modern day living. Our system opens the thoracic cage, stretches the tendons, and facilitates ...." —Joseph Pilates, *New York Herald Tribune*, 1959)

Mr. Pilates met his soon to be wife, Clara, on the boat ride to America. Together, they opened the first Pilates studio in New York City in 1926.

The Awesome Twosome!

Pilates is a stretching and strengthening method that focuses on postural harmony. The ball fits right in and is as versatile as Pilates is. Both methods, as the following list suggests, can teach you how to align your spine and strengthen its supporting muscles.

- Like Pilates, the ball can help correct misalignment in the body.
- Like Pilates, the ball strengthens your postural muscles.
- Like Pilates, the ball can be used to recondition or condition your body—both have roots in rehabilitation.
- Like Pilates, the ball requires that you align your spine when training.

◆ Like Pilates, the ball isolates and strengthens the deep postural muscles so you stand a little taller.

◆ Like Pilates, the ball's shape allows you to train in a reduced stress setting for your joints.

◆ Like Pilates, the ball can be used to recondition and isolate an injury, which helps improve blood flow and speeds up recovery.

◆ Like Pilates, the ball requires good posture; otherwise, you may fall off or loose your balance.

◆ Like Pilates, the ball helps you to develop a sense of coordination, balance, and proprioception.

◆ Like Pilates, the ball is joint friendly because it incorporates similar principles of mobilization and stabilization of the trunk, shoulders, and hips.

Best of all, you can adapt all of Pilates' principles on the ball. In other words, you might recognize the directions and principles if you have been practicing previous ball workouts. If not, don't worry; this chapter covers it all.

From the beginning, my goals were to teach you a little about your body, get you accustomed to working on the ball, and build strength in your body. Although the process may have been long, you can now use what you've learned:

◆ You've learned how to hold yourself, engaging your postural muscles. You should have a fair amount of postural strength along with knowledge on how to tap into this postural power.

◆ You've improved your balance, coordination, and concentration.

◆ You've achieved good overall strength and the ability to stabilize your shoulders, trunk, and hips.

In short, you've already done a lot of hard work. But, unfortunately, if you want to shun that plateau state, you need to create a whole new challenge for your muscles. Pilates on the ball can help burn the fat and transform poochy abs that are resistant to your current training. So, let's get going by memorizing the six guiding principles of Pilates.

On the Ball

The mat exercises were specifically designed to work your muscles in a logical sequence. You won't do many repetitions because Mr. Pilates designed his program to work your muscles synergistically, meaning many muscles at the same time.

The Heart of Pilates

The following six principles define Pilates and form its foundation. They are simple, solid, and make a lot of sense. Pilates engages your mind while working your body, which makes it the ultimate mind and body workout.

1. Concentration
2. Control
3. Centering
4. Flow
5. Precision
6. Breathing

Concentration

"Respect each detail," Joseph Pilates said. Therefore, you must pay attention to every detail of your body. The placement of your head, for example, can make an exercise less safe and efficient. Concentrating is a safety measure that engages your brain while you move your body. In short, you must focus. Some of these exercises are difficult to do especially if your mind is wandering.

Control

Motion without control can lead to injury. Still, haphazard movements can leave you physically hurt and mentally dissatisfied with your performance. As you move your body, first concentrate on what you're about to do and then move with control.

Centering

Pilates and the ball meet where centering begins. Both methods focus on keeping the spine stable before movement in your body begins. Both methods retrain, restore, and realign the natural curves of your spine by strengthening the postural muscles.

Centering strengthens what Joseph Pilates called the *powerhouse*, which is the area of muscles that form your center; it forms a continuous band of muscles wrapping around your waist, from the bottom of your rib cage to your hip bones, and is comprised of your abdominals, back, and hips. In today's terms, this area is often referred to as your core muscles. To find your powerhouse, imagine a huge seatbelt snug across the lower portion of your abdomen, from hip to hip. By centering you'll strengthen your powerhouse or what Joseph Pilates called, "the Girdle of Strength."

Body Ball Language

Powerhouse was the term used by Joseph Pilates to describe the area of muscles that is your center; it forms a continuous band of muscles wrapping around your waist, from the bottom of your rib cage to your hip bones, and is comprised of your abdominals, back, and hips.

Flow

A strong center can lessen the workload on your arms and legs. Once you learn to tap into this internal power, motion can flow from there. After centering, you'll flow from one motion to the next just like you were taught to do in Pilates. Flowing movements look graceful and put less stress on your body.

Precision

Precision makes a difficult exercise look easy. Only after you apply the above principles including the last principle which is breathing to your motions can you focus on precision so your body moves with ease. Your body will become a fine-tuned machine, operating at peak performance while doing these exercises and in your every day life. Practice makes precision— no doubt about it!

Breathing

The final principle is the most important principle: Just breathe! Each Pilates exercise is coordinated with specific breathing instructions. Joseph Pilates suffered from asthma, which is why breath work is the heart of each exercise and is vital to the integrity of Pilates.

I also find great value in it, so much so that I have already asked you to use the lengthened exhalation to activate and strengthen the stabilizing muscles of your spine in earlier ball workouts. This is Pilates at its best!

The *Pilates breath*, also called *lateral breathing*, increases your breathing capacity, enhances the exercises, strengthens your stabilizing spinal muscles, and improves the quality of your life.

Body Ball Language

The **Pilates breath** is very specific and is called **lateral breathing.** You'll inhale through your nose to open your rib cage, laterally. Your belly never rises with this inhalation. You'll exhale deeply through your mouth to purge every last breath from your lungs as if blowing a hundred candles out on a birthday cake. This lengthened exhalation is used to trigger your deep abdominal, the transverse, along with the other stabilizing muscles of the spine.

To laterally breathe, inhale through your nose and float that air to your lungs to open each rib so your rib cage expands laterally. Your belly never rises with this breath. And then lengthen your exhale through your mouth to purge every last breath from your lungs. Your goal is to feel a tightening sensation around your waist to facilitate a contraction of your deep abdominal, the transverse, along with the other stabilizing muscles of the spine.

Try this breath: Put your hands around your rib cage. Inhale through your nose to expand your lateral ribs. Exhale through your mouth as if blowing out 100 birthday candles. Did you feel your ribs expand and your belly pull in? Keep practicing!

On the Ball

Balance requires a joint effort from multiple muscles. Two in particular are adductors and abductors, which co-contract to keep you standing on one leg. When strong, these two muscles co-contract to help you balance in every step you take.

Lateral Breathing Exercises

Why it works: These exercises challenge and strengthen your breath, send your awareness to your stabilizing muscles and strengthen your abdominals. Lateral breathing takes time to master, so use the ball to help increase your breath awareness.

Start/Finish Position

1. Lie on your back with your knees bent.
2. Hold the ball in your hands and then on your belly.
3. Relax and breathe into the ball, lifting the ball to the ceiling.

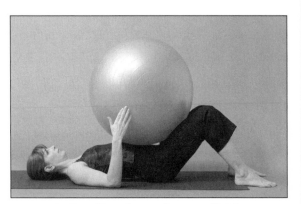

Ball and breath exercise, start/finish.

Movement

4. Now, try your Pilates breath. Inhale into your lateral ribs. The ball should not rise.
5. Exhale deeply so the ball drops toward your spine.

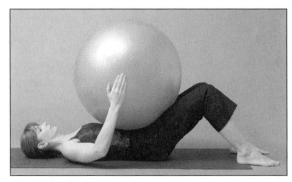

Ball and breath exercise, movement.

The Pilates breath work is vital to the integrity of Pilates. I also think that the Pilates breath can be added to many other exercise programs, including ball workouts.

Pilates on the Ball

Good form is vital in Pilates and keeps you balanced on the ball. As you move closer to a new mind and body challenge with Pilates on the ball, keep in mind these fundamentals:

◆ Maintain a stable (neutral) pelvis. Align your pelvis so it's in a neutral and stable position while doing these exercises. Don't mash your lower back into the mat or overarch. Put your pelvis in neutral.

◆ Lower your ribs to your hips. To strengthen your abs, drop your rib cage to your hips. Your may have a tendency to lift your ribs to the ceiling, which causes your lower back to arch and interfere with your stable spine. Ribs to hips helps engage your trunk's support system, which includes your abdominals, specifically your obliques.

◆ Float your shoulder blades. To help create shoulder stability and strengthen the many muscles of the upper back, float your shoulder blades down your back and keep them there.

◆ Keep your head in line with your spine. Your head is an extension of your spine. Keep it straight. Don't force your chin to your chest or lift your chin to the ceiling. Both positions can displace the natural cervical spine. Always lengthen from the back of your neck.

◆ Engage your deep abdominals by dropping your navel to your spine, which activates your transverse. Navel to spine will help you to stay round in your spine as you roll and unroll.

If this review is completely foreign, see Chapter 3.

The Least You Need to Know

◆ Pilates is a smart strategy to achieving abs, long and lean legs, and a lengthened body with perfect posture.

◆ Joseph Pilates blended a variety of disciplines, from Eastern and Western philosophies, to invent a hybrid mind-and-body fitness method.

◆ Pilates and the ball are similar in fitness elements: Both methods focus on aligning and strengthening your postural muscles, which include the abdominals and back.

◆ Pilates on the ball can help burn fat and transform poochy abs that are resistant to your current training.

In This Chapter

- ◆ New and renew with Pilates on the ball
- ◆ The fab five
- ◆ Fit and fabulous
- ◆ Posture still matters

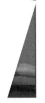
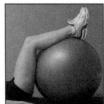
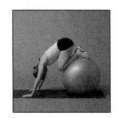
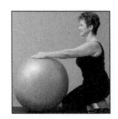
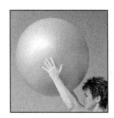
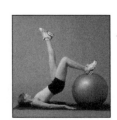

Chapter 8

Mind-Bending Ball Workout

Millions of fitness devotees, many of whom have given up on garden variety workouts, practice Pilates. Why? Because the fitness curious are looking for invigoration, inspiration, and body transformation. So here it is!

The Pilates Plan

This beginner ball mat work adds up to 10 exercises, which is based on the work of Joseph Pilates. Each exercise is perfectly arranged to engage a lot of muscles to work your body in a balanced way. For muscular harmony and body results, do them in order, following all directions and given repetitions. Don't make the mistake thinking more is better; it's not! A well-executed exercise is so much more beneficial to your body than a sloppy one.

Memorize these exercises and run through this mental checklist before moving your body:

◆ Keep your head in line with your spine.
◆ Drop your shoulders.
◆ Pull your belly button up and in.
◆ Stabilize your spine.
◆ Breathe.

Eventually, this checklist will join your mind and body as one, becoming as natural as the exercises themselves.

You can do this mind-bending ball workout every day or as few as two days a week as part of your strength and stretching fitness plan. Don't forget to sweat a little with some cardio. I strongly believe that you need a variety of fitness to keep you and your muscles challenged. So, mix it up and have fun.

The Fab Five

Learning all ten exercises correctly can be overwhelming at first. If you prefer, you can learn the following five exercises first, and then add to them. If that's an option, it may be helpful to photocopy the "fab five" and then place them in the order below creating a mini-guide, so you can memorize them.

- The hundred on the ball
- The Rollup on the ball
- Single-leg stretch on the ball
- Spine stretch on the ball
- Seal with ball

When you're ready to try all 10 exercises, the correct order is below. Keep in mind that the ball makes exercises a little more challenging in general. Pilates is no exception, so listen to your body! You can always drop the ball and just do the Pilates exercises in this order:

1. The hundred on the ball
2. The rollup on the ball
3. Leg circles with ball
4. Rolling like a ball
5. Single-leg stretch on the ball
6. Double-leg stretch on the ball
7. Spine stretch on the ball
8. The saw with ball
9. Side kick ball series (side kick front and back, leg ball circles, ball beats)
10. Seal with ball

On the Ball _____

Joseph Pilates used a long and gradual exhalation as if you're blowing a hundred birthday candles out to trigger the deep muscles of your spine: transversus abdominis, multifidus, and pelvic floors.

The Pilates "V"

Why it works: The Pilates "V" is a traditional stance used in almost every exercise to help stabilize your body and to activate your inner thighs, pelvic floor, and the back of the upper thighs. To feel this contraction, place a small rolled up hand towel between your legs and squeeze it! You might even want to work with the hand towel between your legs at first to help engage this deep inner contraction.

Start/Finish Position

1. Place your heels together and open your feet so your toes are three fingers width apart, making a small "V," and make sure this slight turnout travels the length of your legs, from your hip bones to your toes.

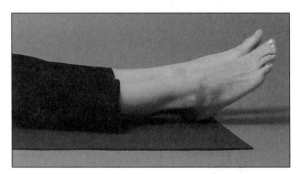

The Pilates "V," start/finish.

The Hundred

Why it works: This classic Joseph Pilates exercise is the first exercise of the mat. The hundred on the ball increases your circulation, warms up your body, coordinates your breath and movement, and challenges and strengthens abdominals.

This exercise requires a fair amount of abdominal strength to maintain proper trunk stability and head and neck alignment. If you have neck strain, don't use the ball. You can also cut the breath work in half, counting to 50 versus 100.

Ball Blowout

If you have any neck strain, please drop the ball. At no time should you work with strain to complete an exercise.

Start/Finish Position

1. Lie on your back.
2. Place the ball between your shins.
3. Stretch your legs to the ceiling, squeezing the ball to keep it in place.
4. Place your arms by your sides, palms down.

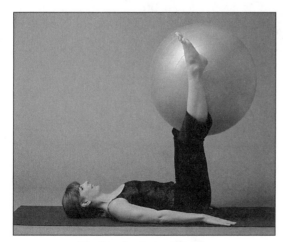

The hundred, start/finish.

Movement

5. Curl your chin to your chest and lift your shoulders off the floor.
6. Place your hands by your sides, palms down.
7. Fingertips reach long as you vigorously pump your arms up and down by your sides while doing the following breath cycles:
8. Inhale for five counts.
9. Exhale for five counts, which add up to ten breaths or one breath cycle.
10. You will complete ten breath cycles to achieve the hundred.

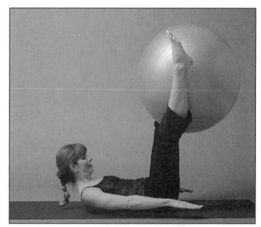

The hundred, movement.

Balancing Ball Tips

◆ If you have a neck injury, please talk to your doctor before doing this exercise.

◆ If you're having a hard time holding your head up, you can reduce the breath cycles to fifty: Inhale for five counts, exhale for five counts, and complete five breath cycles or 50 breaths.

◆ If you can't inhale for five counts, try reducing your breath count. You can begin by inhaling for three counts and exhaling for four counts to ensure that you gradually squeeze all the air out of your lungs. Remember a lengthened exhale is your goal. As your breathing capacity increases, then you can try the traditional breath count as described.

◆ If your back lifts or bounces off the floor, bend your knees and drop the ball to reduce the workload for your trunk.

◆ While pumping your arms, nothing moves except them. Don't bounce your trunk or bob your head. Stabilize your spine by dropping your navel to your spine.

◆ Squeeze the ball to activate and strengthen your inner thighs and pelvic floors.

Ball Blowout

The ball makes an exercise more difficult because it wobbles and forces your abs and back into action. Pilates on the ball is no exception. If you're a beginner or want more detailed information on how to advance in Pilates, consider buying *The Complete Idiot's Guide to Pilates*. This book provides a variety of Pilates workouts for various fitness levels.

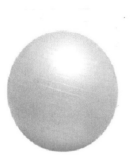
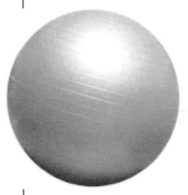

The Rollup

Why it works: The rollup strengthens your abdominals, improves your spine's flexibility, opens and stretches your hamstrings, and sends your awareness to your spine as you learn to peel it off the mat one spinal bone at a time.

Start/Finish Position

1. Lie on your back with your legs extended; feet in a Pilates "V."
2. Place the ball between the palms of your hands and then lift the ball over your head.

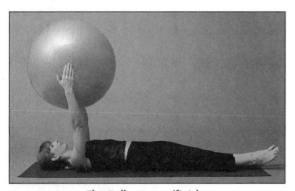

The Roll up start/finish.

Movement One

3. Inhale to lift your chin to your chest and begin to peel your spine off the mat.

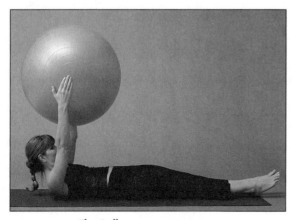

The Roll up movement one.

Movement Two

4. Exhale to lift your shoulders off the mat and round your spine as you curl up.
5. Make sure your feet are in a Pilates "V", to engage your pelvic floor muscles and inner thighs.
6. Round your spine and exhale deeply to pull your navel to your spine, facilitating a deep abdominal contraction as the ball stretches past your toes.

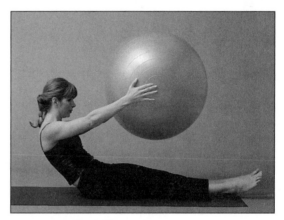

The Roll up movement two.

Movement Three

7. Inhale to tip your pubic bone to the ceiling, feet in Pilates "V."
8. Stretch the ball toward your toes as you squeeze and engage your hamstrings, pelvic floors, and inner thighs.
9. Exhale and press your heels away from your hips.
10. Continue exhaling as you curl down, pulling your belly button to your spine to engage your abdominals to roll down with control, bone by bone.

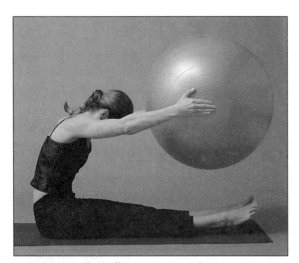

The Roll up movement three.

Ball Blowout

If your abdomen bulges, you are no longer using your abdominal muscles correctly—the rectus abdominus (the most superficial of your abdominals) has become dominant. Try to scoop your belly button up and in under your rib cage to keep your belly from bulging—scoop, scoop, scoop.

Balancing Ball Tips

◆ Don't lift your shoulders; relax them. Slide your shoulder blades down your back to help stabilize your shoulders.

◆ Don't jerk up and drop to the floor. Use your exhalation; slowly uncurl your spine, bone by bone.

◆ If you find it difficult to roll up, drop the ball. Focus on your form and building abdominal strength first by bending your knees and using your hands to guide you up. As you curl down, wrap a towel around your shins and use it to guide you down to the mat.

◆ Imagine a wheel in motion.

◆ Repeat three to five times.

Leg Circles

Why it works: Leg circles tone your hips and thighs, open and nourish your hip joints, strengthen your abs, and challenge your trunk stability. Before leg circles, stretch your hamstrings.

Start/Finish Position

1. Lie on your back with your legs draped over the ball.
2. Press the back of your arms into the mat, palms down.
3. Lift one leg up so your toes reach to the ceiling, toes turned out slightly.
4. Move your other leg so the heel of your foot presses into the ball to hold it steady.
5. Inhale and move the leg that's up toward your nose.

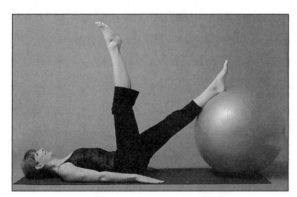

Leg circles, start/finish.

Movement One

6. Exhale as you move your leg across your body, squeezing your inner thighs together.

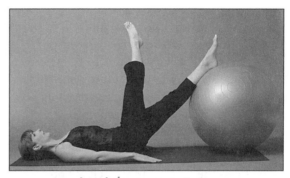

Leg circles, movement one.

Movement Two

7. Still exhaling, circle your leg to the ball.

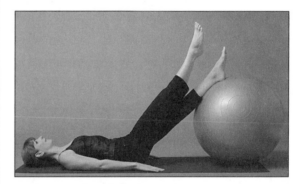

Leg circles, movement two.

Movement Three

8. Still exhaling, circle your leg to the side of your body, and up to your nose.
9. Inhale and pause the motion.
10. Exhale to continue circling your leg.

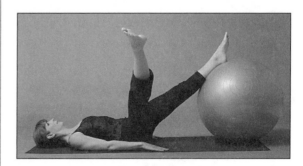

Leg circles, movement three.

Balancing Ball Tips

◆ As your leg circles, it challenges your trunk and pelvic stability. To keep your spine stable, hug your abs to your spine and maintain a neutral pelvis to help off-set the weight of the circling leg.

◆ Try to keep your hips still, no rocking from side to side.

◆ Press the length of the back of your arms, palms down into the floor to help stabilize your trunk.

◆ Keep your circles small. In fact, imagine drawing a circle on the ceiling—emphasize the inner thigh squeeze to tone your thighs and engage pelvic floors.

◆ Both legs are active to help keep the ball from rolling away from you. Stabilize your trunk and pelvis as the ball challenges them.

◆ Press the heel of your foot on the ball into the center of it to help keep the ball still.

◆ Don't rock from side to side as the leg circles—secure your trunk.

◆ Don't lift your chin to the ceiling. If you find that it's hard to rest your head evenly, put a small towel underneath your head to help relax your shoulders.

◆ Repeat five leg circles and then reverse the direction to circle your leg for five.

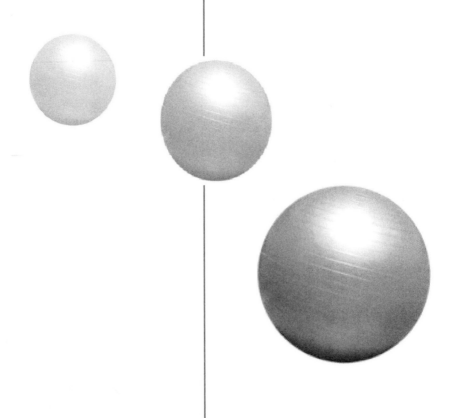

Rolling Like a Ball

Why it works: This exercise improves your digestion and elimination, eases spinal tension, challenges your balance, and strengthens your abdominals.

Ball Blowout

To practice rolling like a ball, you might want to test the water first with a few baby steps:

1. Sit at the edge of your mat.
2. Slide your bottom to your heels.
3. Place the palms of your hands behind the back of your thighs.
4. Tip your pubic bone to the ceiling to lift your toes off the ground, about 2 or 3 inches.

If you're very wobbly, exhale deeply to facilitate the deep abdominal contraction. If you still feel wobbly, don't roll. Practice lifting your toes and then balancing for three to five breaths. Eventually, you'll develop the strength and coordination to roll like a ball.

Start/Finish Position

1. Sit at the edge of your mat.
2. Place your ball on your shins; hold it in place.
3. Lower your chin to your chest and gaze at your belly.
4. Create length in your spine and lift up and over!
5. Lift your toes off the mat, hovering about 1-2 inches.

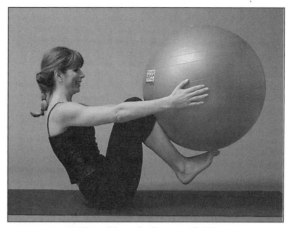

Rolling like a ball, start/finish.

Movement

6. Look at your belly.
7. Tip your pubic bone to the ceiling, scooping your navel to your spine.
8. Inhale and begin to roll back, pressing the ball into your shins.
9. Continue inhaling as you roll to your upper back—your head never touches the mat.
10. Exhale to the starting position.

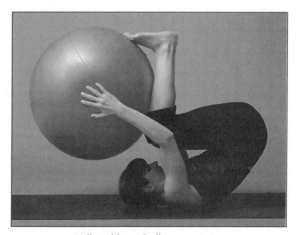

Rolling like a ball, movement.

Balancing Ball Tips

- Don't roll on your neck. Your head must never touch the mat.
- Roll with control. Try not to depend on momentum to roll. Engage your abdominals and pelvic floors by pulling up and in.
- When rolling, your shoulders may lift toward your ears.
- Relax your shoulders.
- Your breath and the roll flow as one motion.
- Repeat 8 to 10 times.

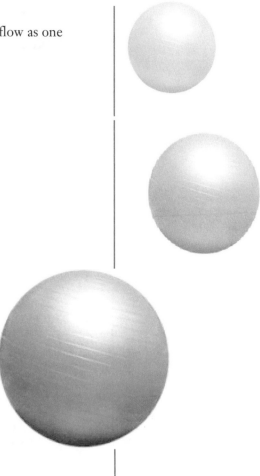

Single-Leg Stretch

Why it works: Single-leg stretch strengthens your abdominals, challenges your trunk stability, and improves your coordination and concentration.

The breath work can be tricky, so let's review it. You'll inhale for two leg stretches meaning you will switch legs while inhaling and then exhale for two leg stretches, switching your legs, which will total one leg stretch.

Start/Finish Position

1. Lie on your back with your right knee bent while the left leg extends.
2. Hold the ball between the palms of your hands and lift it over your head.

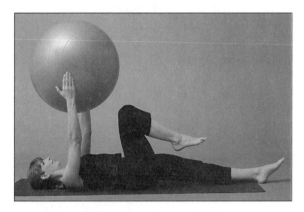

Single leg stretch, start/finish.

Movement One

3. Curl your chin to your chest to lift your shoulders off the mat.
4. Gaze between your thighs.
5. Inhale to lift and then stretch your left leg to the ceiling, keeping toes relaxed and in a natural position

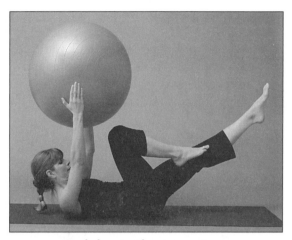

Single leg stretch, movement one.

Movement Two

6. Still inhaling, switch legs so the right leg stretches to the ceiling while your left knee moves to your chest, keeping toes in a natural position.
7. Exhale to switch your legs so your left leg stretches to the ceiling while your right knee moves toward your chest.
8. Still exhaling, switch legs again so the right leg stretches to the ceiling while the left knee moves toward your chest—squeezing every ounce of air from your belly.

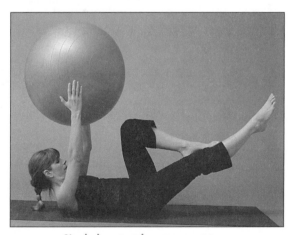

Single leg stretch, movement two.

Balancing Ball Tips

◆ As you switch your legs, stretch your toes away from the hips—imagine miles and miles of legs.

◆ Keep your toes lifted toward the ceiling. When you feel strong enough, you can lower your legs in various levels to continue to challenge your abdominals.

◆ If your neck tires, drop the ball. You can lower your head to the floor and then resume the exercise after a little rest.

◆ Look between your thighs to lengthen the back of your neck.

◆ Your breath is long and gradual so you have enough to alternate your legs.

◆ Don't bulge your belly.

◆ Repeat four to eight stretches alternating with each leg.

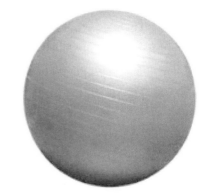

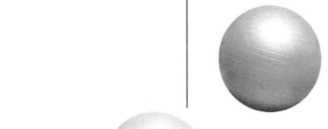

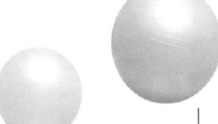

Double-Leg Stretch

Why it works: This exercise strengthens your abdominals, challenges your coordination, and improves your concentration.

Start/Finish Position

1. Lie on your back with your knees bent.
2. Hold the ball between the palms of your hands.
3. Place the ball on top of your shins.

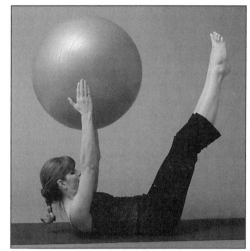

Double-leg stretch, movement.

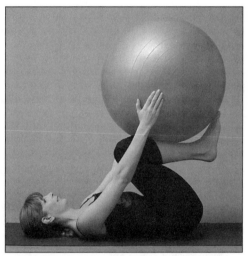

Double-leg stretch, start/finish.

Movement

4. Curl your chin to your chest to lift your shoulders off the mat and gaze between your thighs.
5. Sink your belly to your spine.
6. Inhale to stretch your arms and legs toward the ceiling—the ball moves toward your toes.
7. Exhale to the starting picture—pushing all the air out!

Ball Blowout _____

During the double-leg stretch, your trunk must remain stable. If you feel any tension in your neck, put the ball down. If you still feel neck strain, place a small pillow under your head for support.

Balancing Ball Tips

◆ Don't arch your back. Stay firm and stable in your trunk and pelvis.

◆ Stretch your fingers and toes away from your trunk.

◆ Try to move your arms and legs at the same time.

◆ The breathing rhythm flows like this: Inhale to stretch the ball and legs out; exhale to bring them in, pressing your knees to your chest to empty every ounce of air from your lungs.

◆ As you advance in strength, you can extend your legs a little lower so your toes are in line with your nose, about a 45-degree angle while reaching the ball directly behind and over your head.

◆ Repeat five flowing double leg stretches.

Spine Stretch

Why it works: Spine stretch releases tight back muscles, improves spinal flexibility, develops power in your abdominals as you pull your belly button to your spine, stretches your hamstrings, focuses on stacking each spinal bone, and feels good.

Start/Finish Position

1. Sit on the floor with your legs extended, open about shoulder-width apart.

2. Hold the ball between the palms of your hands, extend your arms in front of you, and pull your belly button in and up while maintaining a neutral spine.

3. Flex your feet to stretch your hamstring, but don't push your knees into the ground.

4. Inhale to prepare for the movement.

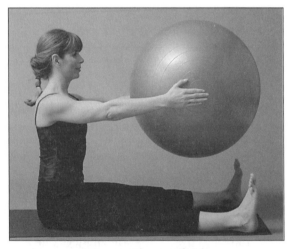

Spine stretch, start/finish.

Movement

5. Exhale to lower your chin to your chest.

6. Continue exhaling as you curl the top of your head toward the floor so your nose lowers between your legs while reaching the ball past your toes.

7. Even though your arms are reaching, pull your belly button up and in so your abs hug your spine, creating a scoop.

8. Inhale to restack your spine, bone by bone.

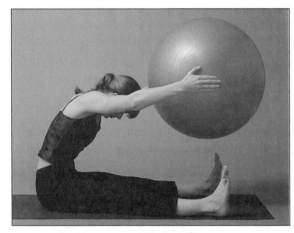

Spine stretch, movement.

Balancing Ball Tips

◆ If your pelvis pulls under, rounding your lumbar spine, your hamstring may be tight. Place a small pad or blanket underneath your bottom to give it a little lift or bend your knees. Your spine should be lifted and straight so as not to put too much pressure on your lumbar (lower back) bones.

◆ Don't move your legs. Focus on rounding over and lifting your navel to the ceiling.

◆ Even though your arms reach to your toes, pull your belly button to your spine so that you can enjoy a deep back stretch.

◆ Relax your shoulders.

◆ Repeat five spine stretches.

The Saw

Why it works: The Saw encourages spinal rotation, tones your spine, stretches tight shoulders and chest muscles, tones your waist, and improves digestion and elimination. In the saw, you'll twist your torso, using your breath to cleanse toxins from your lungs.

Start/Finish Position

1. Sit on the mat and extend your legs, about shoulder-width apart.

2. Press the back of your legs into the mat to help secure your bottom.

3. Sit tall, and find a stable pelvis.

4. Place the ball between the palms of your hands and extend them out in front of you.

5. Inhale to grow taller within your spine to initiate the twist.

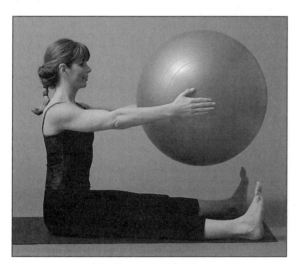

The Saw, start/finish.

Movement One

6. Exhale to turn your chest to the right and place the ball on the opposite side of your right ankle.

7. Continue exhaling as your left hand rolls the ball past your right foot while the right arm reaches behind your back.

8. Imagine pulling your arms apart, reaching your fingertips long to create a deep torso twist.

9. As you lengthen your exhale, use your left hand to roll the ball forward, increasing the intensity of the twist.

10. Drop your left ear toward your right knee and look behind you.

11. Inhale to grow your spine tall and return to the starting picture. Take a deep breath so you have enough air to move into the twist.

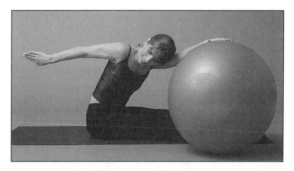

Saw, movement one.

Movement Two

12. Exhale to turn your chest to the left and place the ball on the opposite side of your left ankle.

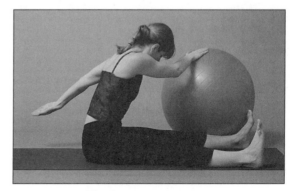

The Saw, movement two.

Movement Three

13. Continue exhaling as your right hand rolls the ball past your toes while the left arm reaches behind your back.

14. Imagine pulling your arms apart, stretching your fingertips long to create a deep torso twist.

15. As you lengthen your exhale, use your right hand to roll the ball forward, increasing the intensity of the twist.

16. Drop your right ear toward your left knee and look behind you.

17. Inhale to grow your spine tall and return to the starting picture.

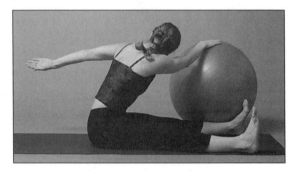

The saw, movement three.

Balancing Ball Tips

♦ Don't bounce in this stretch. Slowly exhale as you deepen your twist, counting to three.

♦ Your legs don't move. The twist initiates from the bottom of your rib cage. Imagine that your legs are glued to the floor.

♦ Deep inhalations and exhalations are necessary to carry you through the complete motions of the exercise: Inhale, growing tall in your spine, and then exhale, counting to one, two, and three to deepen the twist.

♦ The ball is the perfect prop to help deepen your twist and empty your lungs of toxins.

♦ Repeat three to five sets.

Ball Blowout

If you have had a back injury, please ask your doctor if twisting your spine is appropriate.

Side Kick Ball Series: Kick Front and Back, Leg Ball Circles, and Ball Beats

Why it works: This leg series tones your hips, thighs, and butt, opens your hips, and challenges your balance and coordination. All in all, you'll complete three different leg exercises, moving fairly quickly from one to another.

Start/Finish Position

1. Lie on your side over the ball.
2. Bend your bottom leg to help stabilize you and straighten your top leg so only your toes touch the mat.

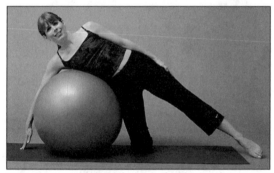

Side kick, start/finish.

Movement One

3. Lift the top leg to hip height. If you feel wobbly, then don't move your leg in the next steps.
4. Inhale to swing your leg forward, kicking two times.
5. Stay solid in your trunk to help keep the ball steady.

Movement Two

6. Exhale to swing your leg back, kicking two times.
7. As the leg swings back, don't arch your back. Engage your abs and glutes, especially during the second small kick.

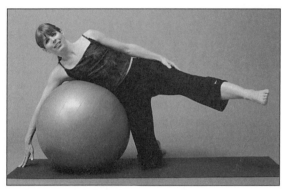

Side kick, movement one.

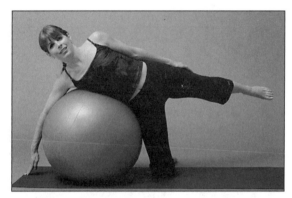

Side kick, movement two.

Balancing Ball Tips

◆ Staying steady in a sideline position on the ball is challenging. You don't have to move your legs forward and back if you're not steady on the ball.

◆ As your leg swings forward, the ball may roll back. Stay lifted and solid in your postural muscles.

◆ Likewise, as your leg swings back, the ball may roll forward. To help secure the ball, pull your belly button to your spine to help prevent your back from arching.

◆ The rhythm for side kick is: Inhale to swing the leg forward, and then quickly add a small kick. Exhale to swing the leg back and then quickly add a small kick.

◆ After six to eight sets, move onto the next exercise, leg circles.

Side Kick Ball Series: Leg Ball Circles

Why it works: Leg circles tone your hips, thighs, and butt, opens and nourishes your hips, and challenges your balance and coordination.

Start/Finish Position

1. Lie in a sideline position on the ball.
2. Bend your bottom leg to help stabilize you.
3. Lift the top leg to hip height.

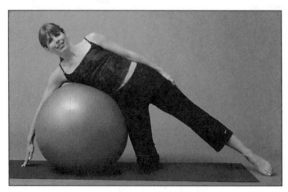

Leg circle, start/finish.

Movement One

4. Inhale to begin the leg circle.
5. Move from your hip bone and circle the leg back to engage your glutes.

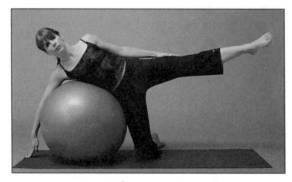

Leg circle, movement one.

Movement Two

6. Still inhaling, sweep your leg to the floor.
7. Exhale to lift the leg to a little higher than hip height to complete the leg circle. If you feel too unstable, keep the leg circles small.

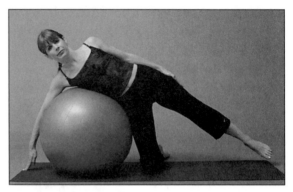

Leg circle, movement two.

Balancing Ball Tips

◆ Be careful! As you move your leg, the ball moves, too. Engage your postural muscles to help keep you steady on the ball.

◆ Circle your leg slowly and make them big enough to tone all of the muscles in your thighs—outer, inner, and butt.

◆ Complete five leg circles and then reverse the direction of the circle.

◆ Without pausing, roll on your belly for ball beats.

Side Kick Ball Series: Ball Beats

Why it works: This exercise tones your butt and inner thighs, strengthens your spinal muscles, develops power in your pelvic floors, and improves your coordination. You'll do two different sets of ball beats to challenge and engage more bottom muscles to de-dimple your derriere: After completing the side kick series on your right leg, do several sets of (quick) ball beats. After completing the side kick series on your left leg, finish with big ball beats. Follow the pictures.

Start/Finish Position

1. Roll on your belly so the ball supports your torso.
2. Place your hands on the floor in front of the ball and gaze at the floor.
3. Lift your legs, engaging your glutes and place your heels together.

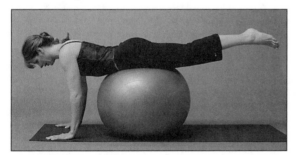

Ball beats (quick), start/finish.

Movement

4. Inhale and click your heels together—quickly, for five counts.
5. Exhale and click your heels together for five counts, which is one set of ball beats. Don't forget to engage your inner thighs, pelvic floors, and glutes.

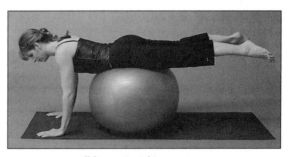

Ball beats (quick), movement.

On the Ball

The side kick ball series is fabulous because you work so many stubborn muscles at the same time. Also great is the fact that your leg movements challenge your core muscles so that they, too, become fit and fabulous.

Balancing Ball Tips

◆ Even though the ball supports your belly, lift the pit of your belly to your spine.

◆ Imagine a thousand dollar bill between your butt cheeks. As your heels beat together, you must hold it in place.

◆ The heel beat rhythm is inhale for 5 heel beats and exhale for 5 heel beats, which is one set of ball beats. You will complete ten sets.

◆ Take a few seconds to drape over the ball and then complete the side kick ball series on the left leg.

You'll finish with big ball beats and reap the same glorious benefits as quick ball beats: a tighter tushie and dimple-free hips and thighs.

Start/Finish Position

1. Roll on your belly so the ball supports your torso.
2. Place your hands on the floor in front of the ball and gaze at the floor.
3. Lift your legs as high as you can, engaging your glutes.
4. Place your heels together.

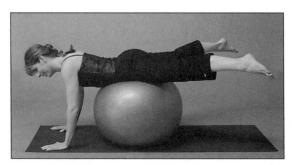

Big ball beats, start/finish and movement.

Movement

5. Inhale to open your legs as wide as you can.
6. Exhale to close your legs slowly to engage your inner thighs, pelvic floors, and glutes.
7. Complete ten sets of big ball beats.

 **On the Ball**

Even though Pilates on the ball is based on the traditional work by Joseph Pilates, both methods challenge and strengthen your postural muscles. This work may take a little time before you feel really comfortable on the ball. But stick with it because the posture payoff is so worth a little ride on the ball.

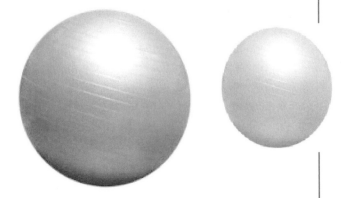

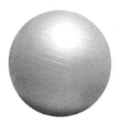

Seal

Why it works: The seal is a spinal treat; it stretches tight back muscles, strengthens inner thighs, and improves balance and control. Seal is classic Pilates exercise that completes your mat workout.

Start/Finish Position

1. Sit on the edge of your mat so your bottom is close to your heels.
2. Open your knees to the side and place the ball between your knees and thighs.
3. Wrap your arms under your legs to reach under your calves so that you can hold the outside of your ankles, with heels together, and gaze at your belly.

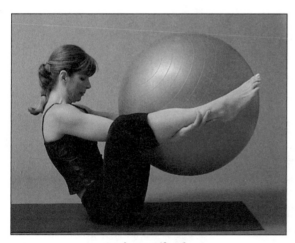

Seal, start/finish.

Movement

4. Lift your feet off the ground about 2 to 3 inches.
5. Inhale to prepare for the movement.
6. Exhale and roll back, lifting your butt cheeks to the ceiling.
7. Don't roll on your head; the bulk of your body weight rests on your upper back.
8. Inhale to roll up—don't lose your ball! Turn on your inner thighs to keep the ball between your legs.

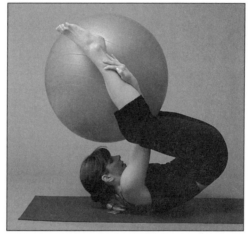

Seal, movement.

Balancing Ball Tips

◆ Don't roll on your head; it never touches the floor. Shift your body weight on your upper back.

◆ Don't throw yourself back into the roll or use lots of momentum. Try to engage your belly and butt muscles.

◆ Gaze at your belly the whole time. Limit your head movements.

◆ Your breath helps you balance so focus on the exhalation when you roll up.

◆ Engage your inner thighs, otherwise you may lose your ball!

◆ Repeat eight to ten times.

◆ Try barking like a seal; it's fun!

The Least You Need to Know

◆ This beginner ball mat workout adds up to 10 exercises, which is based on the work of Joseph Pilates.

◆ The ball makes an exercise more difficult because it wobbles; Pilates on the ball is no exception.

◆ The ball and Pilates blend well because both fitness programs focus on aligning and strengthening the postural muscles.

In This Part

9 Body Ball Therapy

10 Stressed? Then Stretch Over the Ball

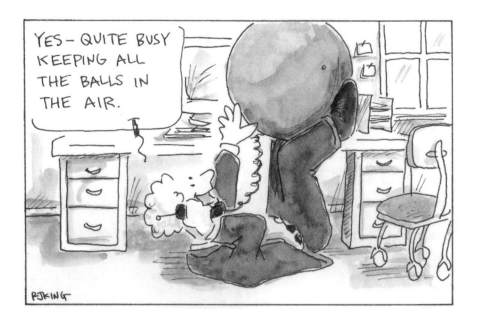

Part 4

Restorative Ball

Got an aching back? Stressed out? Here's your chance to relax, renew, and restore your body with ball exercises. In Chapter 9, physical therapist Karen Sanzo demonstrates the back exercises that she uses to treat back patients. If, on the other hand, you're in need of a stress break, the exercises in Chapter 10 provide relief. Karen and I demonstrate a variety of ball stretches you can even do at work! Not only will you burn more calories, it can ease and erase work tension. Taking a stress ball break is far more beneficial than a coffee break.

In This Chapter

- ◆ Beating the back blues
- ◆ Finding a trained eye
- ◆ Ball is best for reconditioning work
- ◆ Self-diagnosing is dangerous

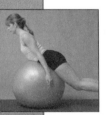 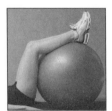 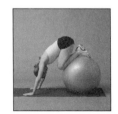 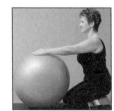 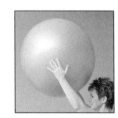 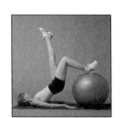

Chapter 9

Body Ball Therapy

Exactly what can a ball do for you? Can it heal a bad back? Can it recondition one after surgery? Can it help keep one healthy?

As of today, many sports medicine physicians, orthopedic surgeons, physical therapists, and chiropractors use the ball to treat various back conditions as an alternative to surgery or as part of a conditioning program after surgery. This chapter specializes in key exercises that have helped individuals recover from the back blues and is, therefore, your anti-aching back campaign.

Back in Business

The good news is "nothing" in life is static. Your condition will eventually change, whether for better or worse. You've got two options: traditional or alternative medicine. Whichever avenue you pick—pharmaceuticals, surgery, or natural healing remedies—you must transform on a whole. Your lifestyle, mindset, physicality, and often your spirit must transform; otherwise, you may end up back where you started.

Today, the ball is used to condition, challenge, and correct the body. Here's why:

◆ With the ball, you can strengthen muscles in a reduced gravity setting and then progress to a gravity challenged setting, while improving the blood flow to all parts of the body to speed recovery.

◆ With the ball, you maintain a crucial balance between strength and flexibility.

◆ You get results because you strengthen your postural muscles.

◆ With the ball, the spine is always addressed—correct posture is a must.

◆ With the ball, you practice coordination, balance, and proprioception.

◆ Each exercise is joint friendly because you incorporate the principles of mobilization and stabilization of the trunk, shoulders, and hips.

The ball can be used to condition or recondition your body because it emphasizes a stable trunk prior to movement of the limbs.

As you now know, the ball teaches you to stabilize your trunk by strengthening sources of stabilization. The abdominals which include the transversus, internal and external obliques, and a variety of back muscles such as the multifidus, erectors, lower trapezius, serratus anterior, latissimus and quadratus lumborum, and rhomboids, plus pulling up through the inner thighs and pelvic floor muscles—or put another way, hip, trunk, and shoulder stabilization! So ball workouts can build strong and yet flexible back muscles and abdominals—especially with the assistance of a trained eye.

Identifying the Trained Eye

With a trained eye, you can use the ball in three ways:

◆ As an option in an attempt to avoid surgery

◆ To recondition the body after surgery or when your physical therapy program is completed and you want to keep up with an exercises program

◆ To rid some of the aches and pains from minor back conditions

Indeed, you can heal yourself! Yes, it's an amazing statement, but the anecdotal evidence is out there to support such a claim. Certain exercises, plenty of body awareness, and of course, good, healthy foods can help heal your body.

I'm not suggesting or advocating self-medication; however, reconditioning on the ball can be another avenue or option to think about and to discuss with your physician or physical therapist before you opt for surgery. Today, many sports medicine physicians, orthopedic surgeons, physical therapists, and chiropractors use or have used the ball as an effective way to build core strength.

The first step is to find a qualified teacher. And I happen to have found one. Karen Sanzo, who is a registered physical therapist and Pilates master trainer (she was one of my Pilates instructors), and I have joined forces to provide you with the latest reconditioning advice.

What exactly do you look for in a physical therapist or a qualified fitness instructor specializing in back injuries?

Obviously, a physical therapist will have a degree from a well-respected physical therapy school. She may have a solid referral base or work at a hospital or orthopedic clinic. Physical therapists or teachers specializing in back reconditioning are often recognized by the sports rehabilitative, orthopedic, and chiropractic communities. For example, some doctors will send patients who are suffering from mild lower back pain to a qualified instructor before taking drastic measures.

Many chiropractors work hand in hand with teachers; some have their own balls set up in their office. Orthopedic surgeons, in addition, may work with physical therapists or teachers that are qualified in the community. These are all good signs that you're choosing a teacher with a trained eye.

You need specialized attention when recovering from back pain, especially since you want to prevent a subsequent episode. You need hands-on guidance so that you work with proper alignment. A trained eye can give you plenty of attention.

Ball Blowout

Watch out for instructors who are not certified or ones who say that they received a weekend certification. Reconditioning work is a specialty that often requires many years of experience or a specific training.

Lumbar Low Down

Your spine is a complex system of interrelated networks consisting of muscle, soft tissue, nerves, and bones. The lower back is the fulcrum for the rest of the body and connects the lower and upper body, which is why, in many cases, the pelvis area influences what the rest of the spine is doing. If, for example, you have an exaggerated curve in the lumbar spine, this can cause imbalances in the hips as well as the thoracic spine.

If the thoracic spine is altered, chances are that the cervical spine is as well, so the downward spinal pain begins. Remember, the body is a closed system; misalignment in one part of the body will eventually affect another part. If, for example, the natural curves of the spine become exaggerated, the bones press down incorrectly on one another creating tension in some muscles while causing weakness in the others. Or put another way, some muscles constantly contract as the opposing muscles weaken. The spinal curves are usually established early in the growing process but can be altered by postural patterns of everyday activities. However, they can also be realigned with corrective and body-friendly exercises.

On the Ball

Lower back problems cost an estimated $50 billion dollars a year in the United States alone in 2000. Back pain is more common than the common cold and is the most frequent activity-limiting complaint in the young and middle-aged. In the industrial world, an estimated 2–5 percent of the population endures chronic aches and many are permanently disabled by them.

Back Matters

Back pain can either be acute (beginning) or chronic (continuous). Sometimes, back woes can be a direct result of poor posture, lifestyle habits that include sports and work patterns such as hunching over a computer. For example, an excessive rounding in the thoracic spine can be caused by long hours hunched over a desk or bent forward to perform your job as a dental hygienist. Likewise, curvature of the lumbar spine can be increased in the third trimester of a pregnancy or carrying a baby in the same arm day in and day out. Dads, too, may develop an exaggeration in the lumbar curve from years of carrying their children.

How, you may be wondering? Let's say that you're eight-months pregnant. The baby's weight can increase your lumbar curve by pushing the hips forward creating a deep arch in the lower back. This shift alters the pelvis so that it rests in an anterior tilt position, throwing your body weight forward and throwing off your body's equilibrium. But because the body is a closed system, the upper back must counterbalance this shift. The thoracic curve rounds forward to help support the baby's weight in an effort to restore your body's equilibrium. Now, you know why back pain is common in pregnancy.

Keep in mind that your lumbar bears your body's weight. Despite being able to handle a wide range of motion—twisting, bending forward and back, and from side to side—your lumbar is vulnerable to injury because it absorbs a lot of stress each day. Muscles, soft tissues, bones, and discs act like the body's shock absorbers. When you run, jump, twist, and fall, this complex network works to protect your spine. As hard wearing as these components are, they will wear out over time if not properly protected and nourished. Therefore, maintaining your natural curves during certain activities and exercises is so crucial to the health of your back. (See Chapter 3.)

Fighting Back the Back Blues

At the very least, an unhealthy spine can leave you miserable. And you have plenty of company if your back aches. Millions of people suffer from constant back discomfort and continue to go through life sticking it out. But don't wait to seek help, because a series of painless micro-injuries can progressively weaken tissues of your body to the point where a mundane everyday activity, such as bending over to pick up something, results in pain or, worse, an injury.

Strain, pain, and injury can strike any time. Ligaments, which connect the bone to the bone, or tendons, which connect muscle to bone, can strain or rip. Muscles that support this system can pull. Joints wear and tear and become arthritic. A bone can break. The delicate discs that are finely balanced between the structure of the bony blocks of your spine can bulge or rupture just by lifting too heavy of an object.

Bones and muscles must work together and be held in place by healthy ligaments, tendons, and cartilage. What could offset this balance? You may have weakened the spinal ligaments and tendons to the point where they can't support your bones and muscles. Structural instability, therefore, makes you more susceptible to improper bone movement and painful misalignment that could, overtime, result in painful conditions such as the following:

◆ Herniated disc. Characterized as a chronic weakening of the outer sheath of the discs. As a result, the gel-like soft contents of the discs bulge through, and press on a nerve exiting the spine causing severe to mild pain.

◆ Degenerated disc. Characterized as chronic weakening to the point where the disc becomes so weak and thin that it can no longer provide a shock-absorbing cushion between vertebrae. As a result, the spinal bones may suffer bone spurs and terribly painful misalignment.

On the Ball

Scoliosis is a condition of the spine, causing lateral displacement in the lower and upper parts of the back; it forms an "S"-like curve in your back. Some people are born with it while others engage in one-sided activities that can alter the spinal curves—for example, professional golfers, tennis players, mothers carrying their babies on the same side, or business executives toting laptops on the same shoulder. Many children can suffer from back pain just by the way they lug their backpacks, especially in the early years of primary development. If you have chronic tightness or dull aching pain, you may want to observe your daily patterns because they could cause muscular imbalance and tightness from one side of the body versus imbalance and weakness on the other. Imbalances between the muscles on the right and left side are common yet not always due to scoliosis. The point is, consider your daily patterns, because with the exception of extreme cases, muscular imbalances from side to side respond very well with body awareness and certain exercises.

Repair and regeneration is greatly dependent on a proper bio-mechanical function. Proper bone alignment, healthy joint movement, strong and flexible muscles, body awareness, and a variety of good, healthy foods that nourish the soft tissues of your body can help heal you.

Don't Get On the Ball

Let's say you felt a "pop" while kneeling down to pick up your briefcase, and you then have a tenderness in your back that doesn't leave. Because you have experienced back pain several years back, you think that you can heal with the exercises you had learned a couple of years ago. So, you buy a ball because you know that strong abs can build a better back.

Diagnosing yourself is downright dangerous. In some cases, the very exercises that you feel may be helping can actually be the ones aggravating your condition. Furthermore, your pain may be caused by something serious, such as a herniated or degenerated disc. If your back pain persists for more than a few weeks or months, or if you have a symptoms such as a muscle spasm that causes you concern, visit your doctor. You don't have to live with pain, especially chronic pain that will eventually compromise your quality of life.

Unfortunately, as great as the ball is, some of you may not be a candidate for the ball. Remember, the ball provides a significant amount of instability even if you are familiar with an exercise. But while this is great for challenging your mind and muscles to new activities, it's not such a good idea to put your body through any additional stress if …

- You're suffering from an acute back pain episode.
- You're suffering from a specific unstable spinal injury or spinal disease that can be aggravated or exacerbated by the ball exercises.
- Your pain increases while using the fitness ball.
- You are fearful of falling in general or don't feel comfortable working on an unstable ball.

Ball Blowout

If your back pain persists for more than a few weeks or months, or if you have symptoms such as a muscle spasm that causes you concern, visit your doctor. If you get the go-ahead from your doctor, you can find a physical therapist or licensed teacher specializing in back conditioning work. Furthermore, this qualified specialist can confer with your doctor to ensure you get the best care possible.

The Fifteen-Minute Back Solution

After months of physical therapy, you're ready to hit the gym. And yet, you're timid about jumping into an aerobics class or lifting weights. That's perfectly understandable!

You can alleviate some minor back pain with patience, a positive attitude, and a daily back and ball workout. So, does that mean you're on your own? Not at all! Make a plan for reconditioning with your physical therapist. You might want to suggest the ball as part of a complete reconditioning plan.

The following series of exercises can provide overall relief and was designed by Karen Sanzo, PT. You might want to bring this workout to your own physical therapist and talk about these exercises, making sure they fit your needs. Ask her to show you these exercises, so you can do them on your own, correctly. Remember, posture awareness enhances any exercise where long-term back remission is your goal. Ask as many questions as you need and take it slow.

- Lower back stretch (subtle pelvic tilts)
- Moving legs with stable spine (feet on ball)
- Hamstring stretch
- Pectoral and latissimus stretch
- Seated spine stretch
- Seated pelvic tilts
- Seated hip flexion, seated knee extension
- Small rotation with neutral pelvis
- Plank (added challenge)
- Raise ball overhead

Ball Blowout

Many people think that their backs are weak, when in fact their backs are overworked.

Lower Back Stretch (Subtle Pelvic Tilts)

Why it works: This is a gentle stretch that relaxes and eases spinal tension in the lower back.

Start/Finish Position

1. Lie on your back
2. Drape both of your legs over the ball.
3. Inhale to prepare for the movement.

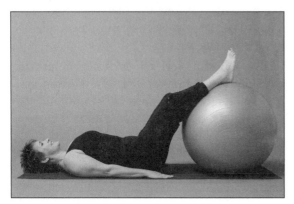

Lower back stretch, start/finish.

Movement

4. Exhale to gently pull your belly button up and in as you curl your pelvis, stretching your lower back.
5. Repeat as many times as you want.

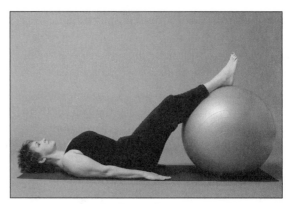

Lower back stretch, movement.

Balancing Ball Back Tips

◆ This pelvic tilt is subtle—don't mash your lower back into the floor.

◆ Use your breath to drop the pit of your belly toward your spine.

◆ Try to relax your back; it's your belly that is working to perform the movement.

Moving Legs with Stable Spine (Feet on Ball)

Why it works: This exercise teaches you to stabilize your spine while your legs move and sends awareness to the back of your thighs while moving the ball out and in.

Start/Finish Position

1. Lie on your back.
2. Drape both of your legs over the ball.
3. Place one foot on top of the ball.
4. Place the other on top of the ball.

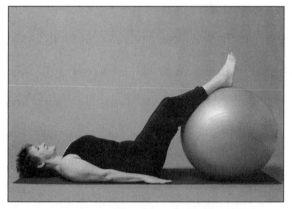

Moving legs with stable spine, start/finish.

Movement

5. Inhale to prepare for the movement.
6. Exhale to pull your belly button up and in and roll the ball toward your bottom.
7. Inhale to roll the ball away from your bottom.
8. Repeat three to five times.

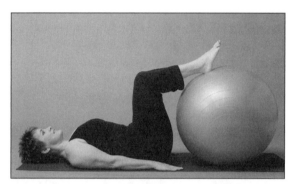

Moving legs with stable spine, movement.

Balancing Ball Back Tips

◆ Relax your back—let the muscles behind your thighs move the ball while the abdominals maintain spine stability.

◆ If you feel any strain in your lower back, reduce the movement. You can make the movement very small at first.

Hamstring Stretch

Why it works: This stretch eases hamstring tightness, stretches the gluteals and relieves lower back pain due to hamstring tightness. In fact, the majority of people with back issues have tight hips.

Start/Finish Position

1. Lie on your back.
2. Drape your legs over the ball.

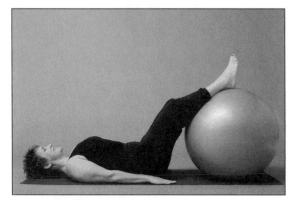

Hamstring stretch, start/finish.

Movement

3. Place your left foot on top of the ball.
4. Move your right leg to your chest and wrap your hands around the back of your thigh.
5. Try to straighten your right leg to the ceiling.

6. Inhale to prepare for the stretch.
7. Exhale to straighten knee and then pull your toes closer to your nose.
8. Repeat three to five times and then change legs.

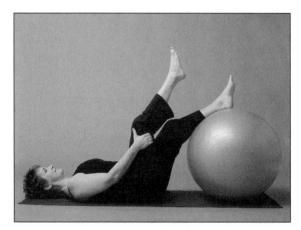

Hamstring stretch, movement.

Balancing Ball Back Tips

◆ The true stretch of the hamstrings is to keep the pelvis in a neutral position and then attempt to lengthen the hamstring.

◆ Keep the hip bones even; it's okay if you can't straighten your leg all the way. In fact, many people can't.

◆ You may want to look for imbalances between the legs—perhaps one is more flexible than the other, which tells you that you favor and work the tighter leg more.

Pectoral and Latissimus Stretch

Why it works: This stretch focuses on lengthening the biggest and most often tightest muscle of your back, latissimus dorsi, while easing tight chest muscles.

Start/Finish Position

1. In a kneeling position, place the ball in front of you and hold it with both hands.
2. Place a rolled up blanket on your heels and sit on it to lessen any knee strain.

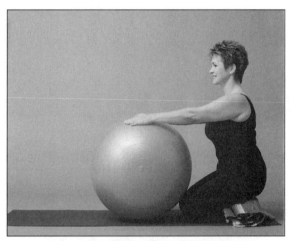

Pectoral and latissimus stretch, start/finish.

Movement

3. Roll the ball out in front of you until you begin to feel a nice stretch.
4. While in position, rest your head on the ball and keep abdominals engaged to stimulate core stability.
5. Breathe naturally and relax tight muscles.
6. Repeat three to five times and then slowly roll the ball in toward your torso.

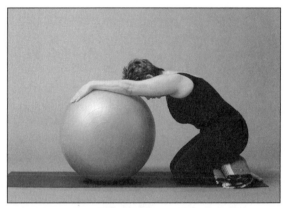

Pectoral and latissimus stretch, movement.

Balancing Ball Back Tips

◆ If you have some upper back or shoulder tightness, you may not be able to rest your head on the ball. Relax your shoulders.

◆ If you can't sit on your heels, place a rolled up blanket between your heels and your bottom.

Seated Spine Stretch

Why it works: This stretch increases flexibility in your back while increasing awareness to the abdominals.

Start/Finish Position

1. Sit on the center of your ball with your knees slightly wider that hip-width, feet parallel and firmly grounded to the floor.
2. Place your left arm behind your back and the right on your belly so you can feel a stable spine.
3. Relax your shoulders.

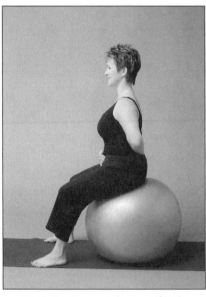

Seated spine stretch, start/finish.

Movement

4. Inhale to prepare for movement.
5. Exhale to lower your chin toward your chest.
6. Continue exhaling to pull your belly button up and in as you continue to round forward, engaging your belly's help to stretch your back.
7. Inhale to slowly straighten each bone of your spine.
8. Repeat three to five times.

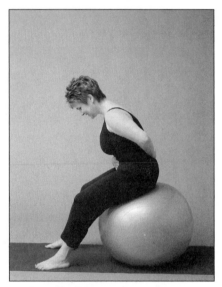

Seated spine stretch, movement.

Balancing Ball Back Tips

◆ Don't mash your chin to your chest. Remember your head is an extension of your spine, so move carefully.

Seated Pelvic Tilts

Why it works: This exercise engages your postural muscles while strengthening and stretching muscles of your lower back and waist. After shifting from side-to-side, return to a neutral position and then shift from front to back to enhance your pelvic awareness and warm up your lumbar spine.

Start/Finish Position

1. Sit on the center of your ball with your knees slightly wider that hip-width, feet parallel and firmly grounded to the floor.
2. Raise your arms so they are parallel to the floor.
3. Relax your shoulders.
4. Relax and take a few breaths to see how your back feels while sitting on the ball.

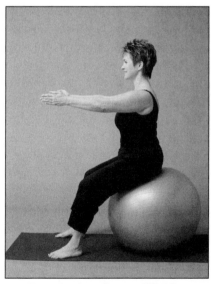

Seated pelvic tilts, start/finish.

Movement

5. Gently pull your belly button to your spine to scoop your belly. Contract your abs and relax your back to get the fullest spine stretch.
6. Return to a neutral position.

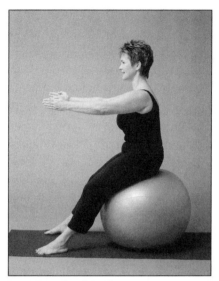

Seated pelvic tilts, movement.

Balancing Ball Back Tips

◆ You're engaging your middle muscles in this exercise, so focus on them.

◆ Don't get frustrated if you scoop your belly without feeling very wobbly. Your back may have been in overdrive, and therefore, your abdominals have weakened. Keep at it.

◆ Don't force the movement; use your abdominal muscles to move the bones of your pelvis.

◆ Relax your back; use your abdominals.

◆ Specifically pay attention to your pelvis. Remember, neutral pelvis is when your pubic bone and two hipbones are in the same line. (See Chapter 3.)

◆ Should any movement cause shooting pain into the buttocks or your legs, stop this exercise.

Ball Blowout

The key to all safe exercising is to feel the belly activation when the spine is stable.

Seated Hip Flexion to Seated Knee Extension

Why it works: This exercise strengthens your postural muscles while you progress from a seated hip flexion to a seated knee extension to actively stretch your hamstrings. This progression challenges your spinal stability as the leg lifts from the floor.

Start/Finish Position

1. Sit on the center of your ball with your knees slightly wider than hip-width, feet parallel and firmly ground to the floor.
2. Place your arms by your sides, and place your hands on the ball for support.
3. Relax your shoulders.
4. As you ground your right foot firmly on the floor, lift your left heel off the ground.
5. Hold this position for five to eight breaths—focusing on maintain the position of your spine and pelvis.
6. Return the heel to the floor and repeat to other leg.
7. If this is challenging for you, then stop here!

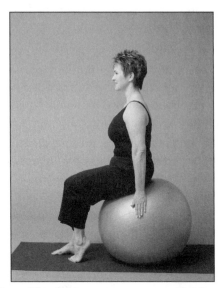

Seated hip flexion movement, start/finish and movement one.

Movement Two

8. Sit on the center of your ball with your knees slightly wider than hip-width, feet parallel and firmly grounded to the floor.
9. Lengthen your arms by your sides, and place your hands on the ball for support.
10. Relax your shoulders.
11. Ground your right foot firmly on the floor.
12. Extend your left knee so the leg is straight only as far as your spine can stay stable.
13. Hold this position for five to eight breaths—focusing on your stable spine and pelvis.
14. Return foot to the floor and then repeat exercise on opposite leg.

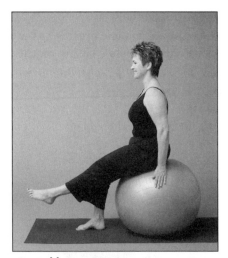

Seated knee extension, movement two.

Balancing Ball Tips

◆ If you feel too unstable lifting your leg, then just lift the heel of your foot. Don't progress to the knee extension exercise.

◆ It's okay for your weight to slightly shift to one side as you pick your leg up. However, focus on keeping your spine and pelvis stable.

◆ Place your hands on your trunk to feel a stable spine and to help you to stabilize: left hand on your back while the right is on your belly.

Small Rotation with Neutral Spine

Why it works: This exercise strengthens your postural muscles while teaching you to keep your pelvis still while rotating your ribs.

Start/Finish Position

1. Place your ball near a wall.
2. Sit on the center of your ball with your knees touching the wall for support.
3. Open your legs so that they are slightly wider than hip-width, feet parallel and firmly grounded to the floor.
4. Lengthen your arms by your sides, and place your hands on the ball for support or on your thighs.
5. Relax your shoulders.
6. Gently press your knees into the wall.
7. Gently turn your bottom ribs to the left without moving your pelvis with your left hand on the ball for support. Hold this position for three to five breaths—focusing on maintaining a stable pelvis.
8. Return to starting position, gently press knees into wall.

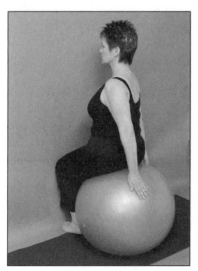

Small rotation, start/finish (back view of the twist).

Movement One

9. Gently turn your bottom ribs to the right without moving your pelvis with your left hand on your knee for support. Hold this position for three to five breaths—focusing on maintaining a stable pelvis.

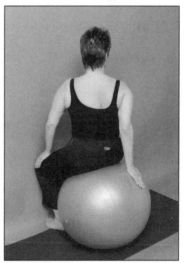

Small rotation, movement one (back view of the twist).

Movement Two

10. Slide your right hand down the ball for support.
11. Turn your chin with the movement only so it's in line with your chest while the pelvis is still.
12. Return to starting position.

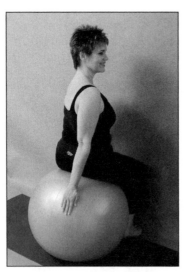

Small rotation, movement one. This picture is the side view of the twist.

Balancing Ball Back Tips

◆ Keep in mind that turning your neck too much won't help you turn your trunk. Keep your chin in line with your breastbone.

◆ As you turn your chest, move from your ribs so the lower back doesn't move. This rotation happens from your bottom ribs, not your lumbar spine.

◆ Press your knees into the ball to keep them even as you turn from the bottom ribs.

 **Ball Blowout**

If the ball is too challenging for you, you can do these exercises on a stool to first learn the movement and build awareness and strength.

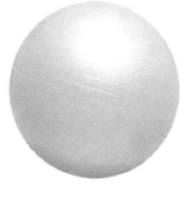

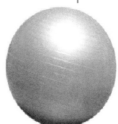

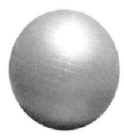

Plank (Added Challenge)

Why it works: The plank builds strength and stability in your trunk and shoulders while teaching you to engage your abdominals in a face down position. This plank is an added challenge for those who feel that they can hold this position without straining their lower back.

Start/Finish Position

1. Kneel in front of your ball.
2. Round your chest, abdomen, and hips over the ball.
3. Place your hands on the floor in front of the ball.

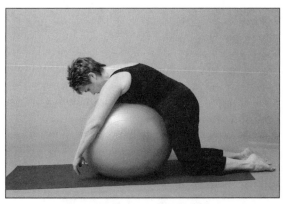

Plank, start/finish.

Movement One

1. Walk your hands out until the ball rolls near your hips and legs are straight.
2. Even though your body is supported by the ball, maintain abdominal and pelvic floor lift for support.
3. Take three to five breaths while maintaining this position.
4. Return to the starting position.

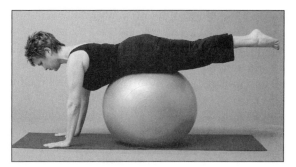

Plank, movement one.

Movement Two

5. Breathe, relax, and drape yourself over the ball.

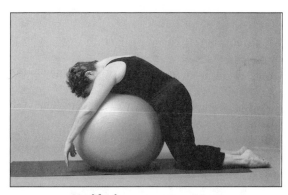

Modify drape, movement two.

Balancing Ball Tips

◆ Ideally, pulling the pit of your belly to your spine should be a gentle action—not forced so that you feel any tension in your lower back.

◆ Proper hand placement is a must for training upper back and shoulder muscles correctly: Your hands are directly under your shoulders. As you slide your shoulder blades down your back, this will prevent your shoulders from elevating toward your ears.

◆ If you experience lower back strain, first check your alignment. Perhaps you're not engaging your abdominals, or your hands are too far from the ball. If pain persists, stop this or any exercise.

Raise Ball Overhead

Why it works: This exercise teaches you to move your arms and keep your spine stable plus it's a feel-good way to end this routine as you roll through your spine.

Start/Finish Position

1. Stand in front of your ball.
2. Bend over to hold your ball in your hands and bend your knees slightly.

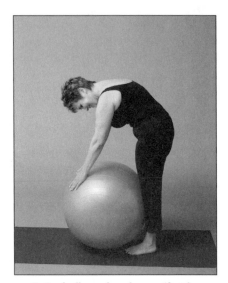

Raise ball overhead, start/finish.

Movement One

3. Inhale to prepare for the movement.
4. Exhale to lift the pit of your belly up and in toward your spine and begin to roll the ball up your body.

Movement Two

5. Breathe normally as you lift the ball over your head, being careful not to lean back.
6. Complete three sets and give yourself a big hug for a job well done.

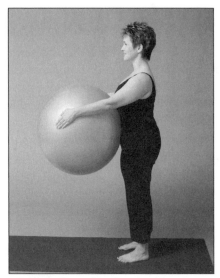

Raise ball overhead, movement one.

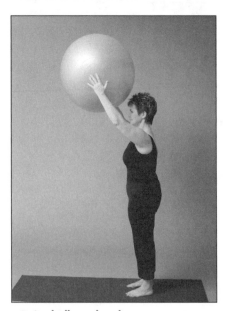

Raise ball overhead, movement two.

Balancing Ball Back Tips

◆ When you contour your body with the ball, try rolling down the ball slowly—it feels good.

◆ While standing to lift the ball over your head, keep your shoulders in line with your hips without leaning back.

◆ Relax your shoulders even as you lift the ball over your head.

Lasting Therapy

One last thought. The following list of guidelines will help you to avoid injury in the first place:

◆ Always focus on the body's optimal biomechanical structure: Focus on accurate bone alignment and proper joint movement.

◆ Nourish your body with nutrients that regenerate connective tissues such as cartilage, ligaments, tendons, and muscles.

◆ Exercise regularly. Movement is essential to delivering precious nutrients to and removing waste products from the cells in your body.

◆ Reduce stress and get your sleep to regenerate your body.

◆ And drink a lot of water.

The Least You Need to Know

◆ Ball exercises can recondition your back.

◆ Today, many sports medicine physicians, physical therapists, and chiropractors use the ball as means for core conditioning.

◆ Ball and back workouts focus on strengthening your postural muscles.

◆ If your back pain persists for more than a few weeks or months, or if you have symptoms such as muscle spasms or radiating pain that cause you concern, visit your doctor.

In This Chapter

- ◆ Restorative ball
- ◆ Sooth your soul
- ◆ Muscle Relief
- ◆ Take your ball to work

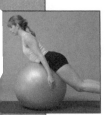 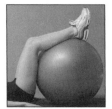 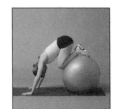 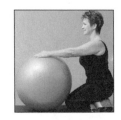 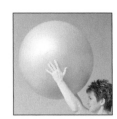 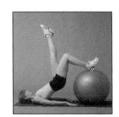

Chapter **10**

Stressed? Then Stretch Over the Ball!

To balance your body and your life, you need to turn within and study your imbalances. If you eat too much, your body shows you. If you work long hours, sacrificing sleep, your body gets sick. If your muscles are tight or weak, your body aches. Sometimes, symptoms are subtle while others can sideline you. Nevertheless, precious moments are stolen from your life.

To look inward takes nothing less than the courage to speak the truth about what is happening in your body and the ability to say "no." To find balance, you have to walk that fine line between too much and too little. Often, this inner dialogue begins as you sit, absorbing quiet time to open blocked channels whether emotional or physical.

So close the door, turn on your favorite inspiration music, light a candle, and breathe. These restorative stretches slow you down so you can sit quietly to explore imbalances in your body and your life.

Renew, Relax, and Restore

Muscle tightness can leave you unbending and unbearable. In some cases, muscle imbalance can alter your alignment setting off the downward spiral that can lead to injuries. If for example, tendons, ligaments, and muscles shorten, the range of motion of the corresponding joint is often restricted as well.

Stretching can counter tightness by lengthening muscles and the soft tissues, which can also help your joints maintain a natural range of motion. Stretching is the best thing you can do to help restore and maintain musculoskeletal integrity, which is why stretching is an essential component of fitness; it enhances your quality of movement.

On the Ball

If you incorporate strengthening and stretching exercises into your healing process, you'll heal faster. In fact, people who stretch have fewer injuries and heal quicker.

Restorative Ball

The shape of the fitness ball makes the perfect prop for stretching in a variety of positions. The ball is especially beneficial if your range of motion is limited. If, for example, you have trouble getting on and off the floor, you can sit on the ball and still stretch tired muscles. The following are a few other benefits of restorative ball:

◆ Your muscles must work to stabilize you. Therefore you can enjoy both stretching and strengthening benefits.

◆ You can maneuver your body in a variety of positions. Because the base of the ball lifts you off the floor, you can get stretching benefits while sitting on the ball, which provide a nice option for people who have trouble getting on and off the floor.

◆ You have more positions, and therefore, more opportunity to deepen your stretch than you would on the floor.

◆ The majority of your body weight is supported, reducing stress to certain joints in your body.

◆ You can arch or round over the ball and enjoy a full spinal length stretch. Spinal traction reduces compression and encourages spinal muscles to relax.

◆ You still challenge your balance and increase your concentration and coordination.

The Restorative Plan

To renew and restore balance to your body, you'll stretch each primary muscle group for no less than one to two minutes (10–15 deep breaths) for the stretches listed in the following pages. You can stretch after the ball workouts in this book to decrease post-exercise soreness and lengthen the muscles you've just shortened. Or, feel free to stretch after your cardio workouts as part of a relaxing cool down. Honestly, you can use these stretches whenever you need to sooth your soul. And you can do this at work as well. That's right, take your ball to work and stretch at your desk for a mini-stress break.

For these stretches, you need one- or two-pound dumbbell weights and a yoga strap. Do these stretches two–three times a week as part of a balanced weekly workout program.

On the Ball

Why not bring the ball to work with you? You can sit on the ball and tone your torso while typing away at your desk. Sounds efficient? It is. Just think about all those extra calories you can burn by recruiting more muscles than just sitting in an office desk chair.

Seated Neck Stretch

Why it works: This stretch soothes frazzled nerves, relieves pent-up stress in your neck and shoulders, and provides a deep stretch for tight neck muscles.

Start/Finish Position

1. Sit on the center of your ball with your knees slightly wider than hip width, feet parallel and firmly grounded to the floor.

2. Hold a dumbbell in each hand, and place your arms at your sides.

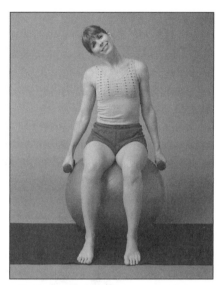

Seated neck stretch, movement one.

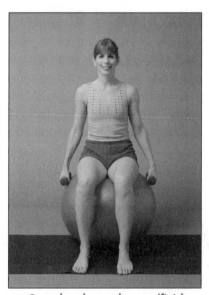

Seated neck stretch, start/finish.

Movement One

3. Slowly lower your right ear to your right shoulder. The weight of your head and gravity deepens the stretch of your neck while the dumbbell weight drops your opposite shoulder.

Movement Two

4. Slowly lower your left ear to your left shoulder. The weight of your head and gravity deepens the stretch of your neck while the dumbbell weight drops your opposite shoulder.

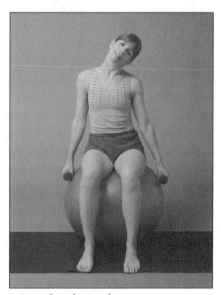

Seated neck stretch, movement two.

Balancing Ball Tips

◆ If you have a neck or shoulder injury, please talk to your doctor before stretching.

◆ Your postural muscles are active to keep your spine stable.

◆ When moving your head from ear to ear, slowly guide it into place.

Seated Back Stretch

Why it works: This stretch eases muscle fatigue and releases the back muscles including spinal erectors, trapezius, and rhomboids.

Start/Finish Position

1. Sit on the center of your ball with your knees wider than your hips, feet parallel and firmly grounded to the floor.
2. Straighten your arms by your sides.

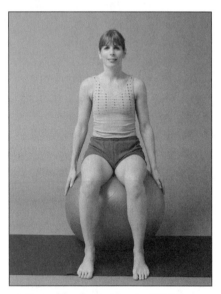

Seated back stretch, start/finish.

Movement

3. Interlace your fingers and place your hands in front of you. Lift your arms to chest height, and rotate your hands so the palms of your hands face out.
4. At the same time, pull your belly button to your spine and roll the ball forward, rounding your spine.
5. Return to neutral spine, sitting on the center of your ball.

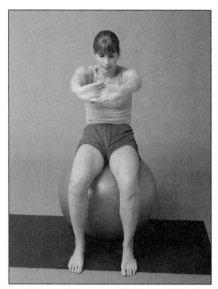

Seated Back Stretch Movement.

Balancing Ball Tips

- This stretch also turns your hands around so you may feel a nice opening within each finger.
- With every exhale, pull your belly button to your spine to deepen the back stretch.

Ball Blowout

Even though seated stretches on the ball are a great option for people having a hard time getting on and off the floor, the ball still wobbles, so there is an added balance challenge.

Seated Chest Stretch

Why it works: This stretch restores length to very tight chest and shoulder muscles. When tight, these muscles can permanently round your shoulders forward. You can lose an inch in height while your breathing becomes restricted.

Movement Two

1. Sit on the center of your ball with your knees wider than your hips, feet parallel and firmly grounded to the floor.
2. Place your hands behind your back and interlace your fingers, palms of your hands together, if possible.
3. Lift your arms, slightly, and at the same time roll the ball slightly behind yourself to arch your spine.
4. Lift the pit of your belly to your spine for support.

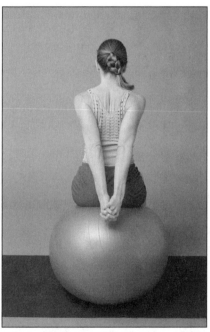

Seated chest stretch, movement two.

Balancing Ball Tips

◆ Before stretching, lift your shoulders to your ears and then slide your shoulder blades into their pockets on your spine.

◆ Shoulder and chest tightness may prevent you from closing the palms of your hands or lifting your arms. Take it slow!

◆ Gently lift your arms with every breath you take.

Pectoral Stretch

Why it works: This stretch lengthens your pectorals and opens your chest.

Start/Finish Position

1. Kneel in front of your ball.
2. Hold your ball with your right hand, palm down.
3. Place your left hand on the floor, palm down.

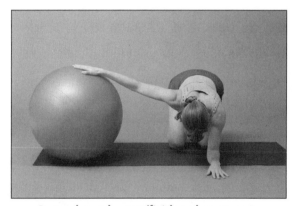

Pectoral stretch, start/finish and movement.

Movement

4. Bend at the waist to roll the ball away from your body.
5. Stack your hips over your knees.
6. Roll the ball to the side and away from your body.
7. Align your hips over your knees.
8. To deepen the stretch, roll the ball out even more.

Balancing Ball Tips

◆ Keep your hips even and stable so you can focus on the upper body stretch.

◆ You can sit on your heels if that is more comfortable for you.

Seated Rotation Stretch

Why it works: This twist soothes frazzled nerves, cleanses your organs, and lengthens tight back muscles.

Start/Finish Position

1. Sit on the center of your ball with your knees slightly wider than hip-width apart, feet parallel and firmly grounded to the floor.

2. Move your right arm over your left thigh, palm up. Place your left arm behind your back so your hand touches the ball for support.

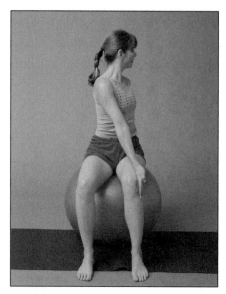

Seated rotation, movement.

Balancing Ball Tips

♦ It's very important that you inhale to grow tall in your spine and then exhale to twist.

♦ Imagine squeezing your lungs of its impurities with each twist.

♦ Don't turn your lower body as you twist. Try to maintain a stable pelvis so your hips don't shift.

♦ Drop your shoulders.

♦ Your head follows the line of your spine.

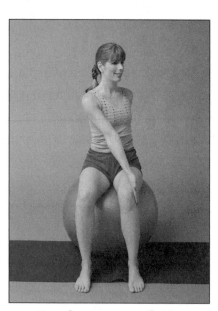

Seated rotation, start/finish.

Movement

3. Inhale to grow tall in your spine, from the top of your head.

4. Exhale to twist your torso to the left.

5. At the same time use your right arm as leverage against your left thigh to deepen the twist until you look over the left shoulder.

6. Repeat to left side.

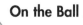

On the Ball

Twist, churn, cleanse, and remove toxins and tension from your back and abs. Imagine releasing the spinal muscles while cleansing your abdominal organs.

Seated Lateral Trunk Stretch

Why it works: This side bend stretches the muscles on the side of your body including your breathing muscles, the intercostal muscles of the rib cage.

Start/Finish Position

1. Sit on the center of your ball with your knees wider than your hips, feet parallel and firmly grounded to the floor.
2. Straighten your right arm to the ceiling and then overhead, lengthening past your ear.
3. Place your left hand on the ball for support.

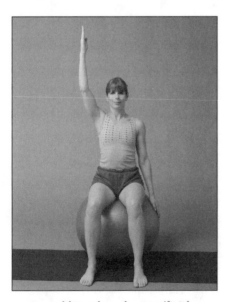

Seated lateral trunk, start/finish.

Movement

4. In one motion, inhale to lift and lengthen your right fingers to the ceiling and then move your arm over your head and past your ear.
5. Hold the ball for support with your left hand because it may roll as your deepen the stretch.

6. Look forward as you deepen the stretch of your right side of your spine with every exhale.
7. Repeat to the other side.

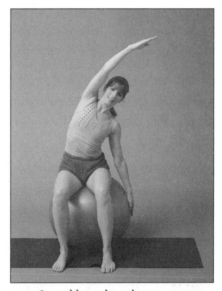

Seated lateral trunk, movement.

Balancing Ball Tips

◆ It's important to lengthen the fingertips to the ceiling first and then stretch over. Always lengthen before stretching laterally.

◆ If you feel very secure on the ball, you can take the opposite hand and place it on your thigh to deepen your side stretch.

◆ Even though your hand is lifted, try to relax your shoulders.

On the Ball

Side bends lengthen and stretch the intercostal muscles and enhance rib cage movement, which can be restricted because of tightness, from poor posture to lack of stretching in the first place. Flexible intercostal muscles help improve your breathing and add freedom of movement to your rib cage.

Supine Arm Circles

Why it works: This stretch opens your shoulder joints, plus stretches all the muscles of your shoulders and upper back.

Start/Finish Position

1. Sit on the center of your ball and walk down the ball so your back drapes over the ball with your head on the ball.

2. Extend your legs out in front of you.

3. Place a very light dumbbell (one to two pounds) in each hand.

4. When you are secure on the ball, extend your arms to the ceiling, knuckles in.

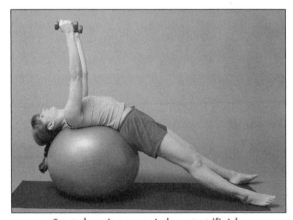

Seated supine arm circles, start/finish.

Movement One

5. Inhale to lower your arms behind you, knuckles in.

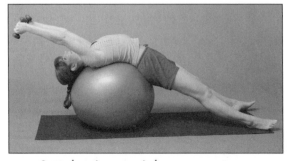

Seated supine arm circles, movement one.

Movement Two

6. Exhale to circle your arms to the sides of your body, palms up.

7. Still exhaling, complete your arm circle by lengthening your hands to the ceiling.

8. Repeat three to five circles and then reverse the circles.

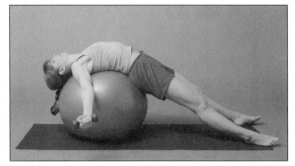

Seated supine arm circles, movement two.

On the Ball

Supine stretch over the ball opens your heart and quiets your mind. Use your breath to open tight areas in the front of your body, especially the muscles that make up your posture, such as chest and shoulder muscles.

Balancing Ball Tips

◆ Please use light weights or no weights because your shoulder joints are delicate.

◆ Don't forget to use your breath to increase the stretch and let go of stress: Inhale to initiate the circle and exhale to finish the arm circle.

Hamstrings Stretch

Why it works: This stretch lengthens your hamstrings and eases tension in your back.

Start/Finish Position

1. Lie on your back.
2. Place your left heel on the ball, so your knee faces the ceiling.
3. Move your right knee to your chest and wrap a yoga strap around the sole of your foot.
4. Straighten your right leg.
5. Inhale to prepare for the movement.
6. Exhale to move your toes closer to your nose.

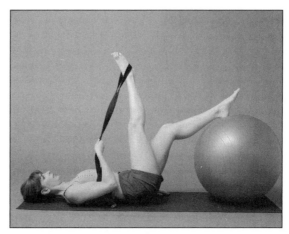

Hamstrings stretch, movement one.

Movement Two

9. Inhale to prepare for the movement.
10. Exhale to move the leg away from your body.

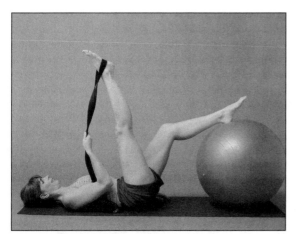

Hamstrings stretch, start/finish.

Movement One

7. Inhale to prepare for the movement.
8. Exhale to move your right leg across the midline of your body.

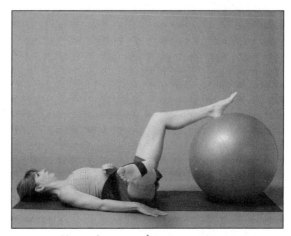

Hamstrings stretch, movement two.

Balancing Ball Tips

◆ Keep your hip bones even and stable. This is vitally important to lengthening your hamstrings correctly.

◆ Try to straighten your leg, but if you can't, that's okay. Focus on maintaining a neutral pelvis.

◆ Use the yoga strap to increase the intensity of the stretch.

Spinal Twist

Why it works: This twist eases tight back muscles and stretches your chest and shoulder muscles in a reduced gravity setting.

Start/Finish Position

1. Lie on your back with your knees bent.
2. Place the ball between your hands.
3. Lift the ball over your head.

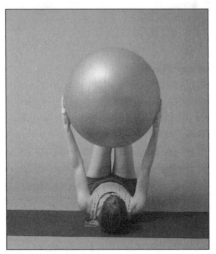

Spinal twist, start/finish.

Movement One

4. Inhale to prepare for the movement.
5. Exhale to turn your knees to the right as the ball moves to the left, twisting your torso.
6. Relax and enjoy this stretch.

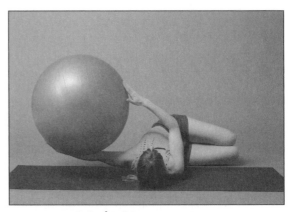

Spinal twist, movement one.

Movement Two

7. Inhale to prepare for the movement.
8. Exhale to turn your knees to the left as the ball moves to the right, twisting your torso.
9. Relax and enjoy this stretch.

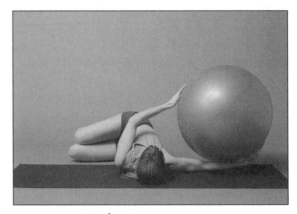

Spinal twist, movement two.

Adductor Stretch

Why it works: This stretch opens and lengthens deep adductors and groin muscles.

Start/Finish Position

1. Lie on your back with your ball close to your bottom.
2. Place the soles of your feet on the ball.
3. Lengthen your arms by your sides.

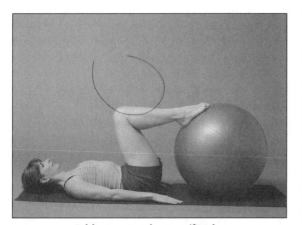

Adductor stretch, start/finish.

Movement

4. Open your knees so the soles of your feet touch.

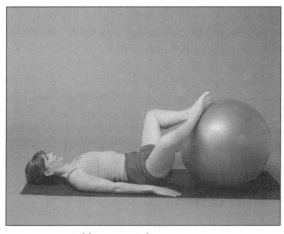

Adductor stretch, movement.

Lower Back Stretch

Why it works: This stretch eases spinal tension and releases tight overused back muscles such as erector spinae.

Start/Finish Position

1. Lie on your back with your legs draped over the ball, which should provide a nice stretch.
2. Lengthen your arms by your sides.

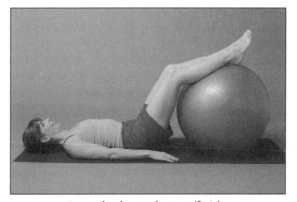

Lower back stretch, start/finish.

Movement

3. Gently tilt your pubic bone to the ceiling to scoop your navel to your spine.
4. Return to neutral.

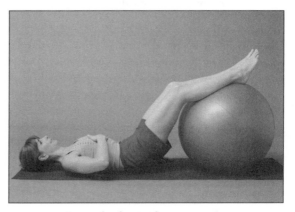

Lower back stretch, movement.

Gluteal Stretch

Why it works: This stretch relieves hip tension and lengthens the outer portion of your thighs and gluteals.

Start/Finish Position

1. Lie on your back with your ball close to your bottom.
2. Drape your legs over the ball.
3. Place your arms at your side.

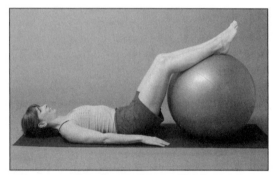

Gluteals stretch, start/finish.

Movement

4. Cross your right ankle over your left thigh and let your knee fall toward your shoulder.
5. Roll your ball toward your bottom with your leg on the ball to increase the outer thigh and gluteals stretch.

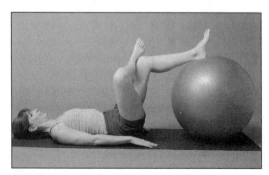

Gluteals stretch, movement.

Thread the Needle Stretch

Why it works: This stretch eases upper back tension and lengthens your latissimus and rear deltoids.

Start/Finish Position

1. Kneel in front of your ball.
2. Hold your ball with both hands, palms down.

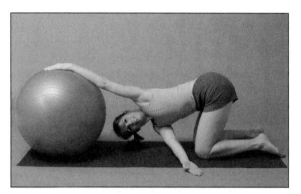

Thread the needle stretch, start/finish and movement.

Movement

3. Bend at the waist to roll the ball away from your body.
4. Keep your hips over your heels.
5. Cross your right hand underneath the left shoulder don't shift your knees.
6. Roll the ball away from your torso to deepen the stretch as you reach your arm underneath your shoulder.
7. Repeat with opposite arm.

Sideline Stretch

Why it works: This stretch lengthens the muscles of your side and makes your spine flexible.

Start/Finish Position

1. In a kneeling position, place the ball against your right hip and thigh.
2. Place your right hand on the ball and extend your left arm to the ceiling, palms in.
3. Drape over ball to further stretch your spine.

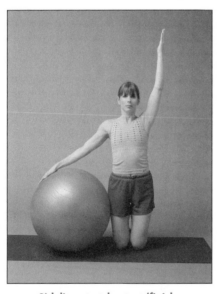

Sideline stretch, start/finish.

Movement

4. Inhale to lift and lengthen your fingertips to the ceiling.
5. Exhale to lean over the ball to enjoy a stretch on the left side of your body.
6. Repeat to opposite side.

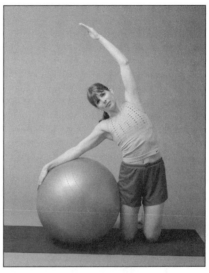

Sideline stretch, movement.

Prone Quadriceps Stretch

Why it works: This stretch lengthens the muscles of the quadriceps and opens tight hips due to overuse.

Start/Finish Position

1. Kneel in front of your ball.
2. Round your abdomen and hips over the ball, so you're facedown.
3. Place your hands on the floor in front of the ball.

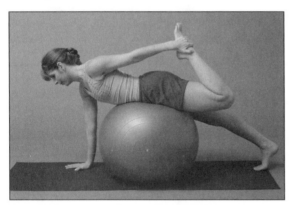

Quadriceps stretch, start/finish and movement.

Movement

4. Lift your right hand off the floor and bend your right knee so your right hand can hold the front part of your foot.
5. Press your foot into the palm of your hand to increase the stretch for the thigh.
6. Repeat other leg.

Balancing Ball Tips

◆ The bones of your pelvis should be even.
◆ Don't twist your knee to the side to hold your foot or shin to achieve the stretch. If you can't reach your foot or shin, try wrapping a yoga strap around the front of your foot.
◆ Contract your buttock muscles to deepen the quadriceps stretch.

Supine Spinal Traction

Why it works: This stretch increases flexibility in your back, prevents back pain, opens tight chest and shoulder muscles, and stretches your abs; it's also a mild backbend so you may feel invigorated!

Start/Finish and Movement

1. Sit on the center of your ball and walk down the ball so your mid-back presses into the ball.
2. Arch over the ball—letting each bone of your spine melt into it.

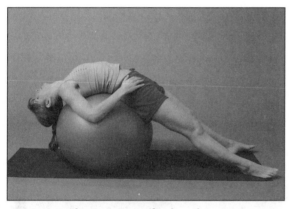

Supine spinal traction, start/finish and movement one.

Movement

3. Extend your legs in front.
4. Place your hands on your hips.
5. Your head is supported by the ball.

Balancing Ball Tips

◆ If you have a back injury, please leave this stretch out.

◆ You can hold a very light pair of dumbbell weights in each hand to increase the chest stretch.

◆ If you're not accustomed to arching, you may experience some dizziness especially when you come out of the stretch. Please rise slowly.

Seated Buttocks and Hamstrings Stretch

Why it works: This stretch lengthens your hamstrings and buttock muscles plus eases tension in your back from sitting at your desk for many hours.

Start/Finish Position

1. Sit on the center of your ball and straighten your legs in front of you, about hip-width apart, toes face forward. Hands rest on your thighs.

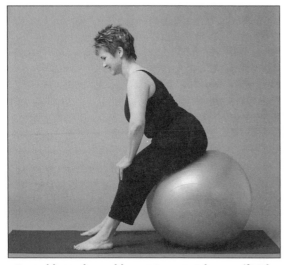

Seated buttocks and hamstrings stretch, start/finish.

Movement One

2. With a straight spine, lean forward and straighten your legs as much as possible. At the same time, the ball will roll behind you.

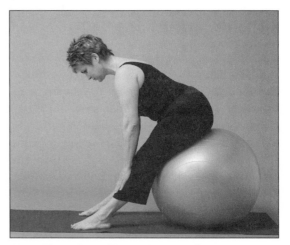

Seated buttocks and hamstrings stretch, movement one.

Movement Two

3. To deepen the stretch, round your spine.
4. Drop your head toward the ball and gaze at it.
5. Interlace your arms behind your calves.

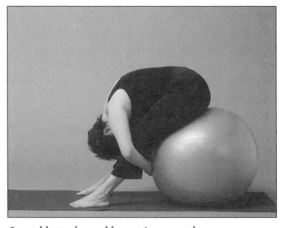

Seated buttocks and hamstrings stretch, movement two.

Balancing Ball Tips

◆ Don't hyperextend your knees. Your legs are straight, but you should not feel any pain in the back of the knee.

◆ Just relax every muscle in your upper back.

Standing Shoulder Stretch at Wall

Why it works: This stretch relieves work-related tension in your shoulders and upper back.

Start/Finish

1. Place the ball on the wall.
2. Stand in front of the ball, a comfortable arm-width distance.

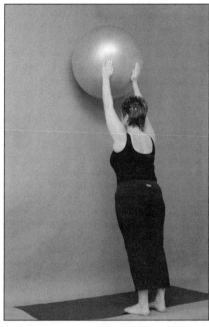

Standing shoulder stretch at wall, start/finish and movement.

Movement

3. Roll the ball up the wall.

Balancing Ball Tips

◆ Just relax and let the ball deepen your stretch as it rolls up the wall.

◆ If you have a shoulder injury, this stretch may not be appropriate for you.

Standing Back Stretch

Why it works: This stretch lengthens and rounds your entire spine to ease tension.

Start/Finish

1. Hold your ball in both your hands and place it on your thighs.

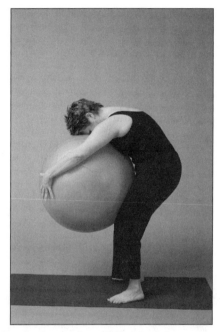

Standing back stretch, start/finish and movement.

Movement

2. Round over so you feel a lengthened stretch in your spine.

Balancing Ball Tips

◆ Take a little time to indulge during your day to relieve nine to five stress so you can leave it at the office.

Seated Neck Stretch

Why it works: This stretch relieves tension in your neck and shoulders, plus it provides a much-needed stretch for your tight neck muscles.

Start/Finish Position

1. Sit on the center of your ball with your knees wider than your hips, feet parallel and firmly grounded to the floor.

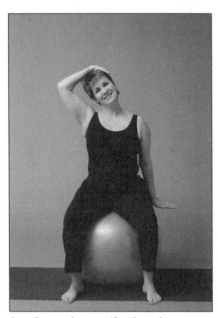

Seated neck stretch, start/finish and movement one.

Movement

2. Slowly lower your right ear to your right shoulder.
3. Press your left palm toward the floor to deepen the stretch.
4. Repeat to the left side.

Balancing Ball Tips

◆ If you have a neck or shoulder injury, talk to your doctor before stretching.

◆ Your postural muscles are still active while maintaining a neutral spine.

◆ When moving your head from ear to ear, slowly guide it in place.

Supine Spinal Traction

Why it works: This stretch increases spinal flexibility and most important, opens and stretches tight chest and shoulder muscles, which have a tendency to round forward as you sit at your desk.

Start/Finish Position

1. Sit on the center of your ball and walk down ball so your mid-back presses into the ball.

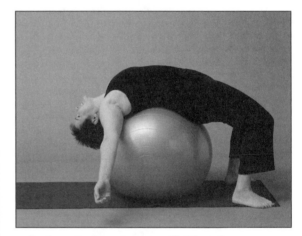

Supine spinal traction, start/finish and movement.

Movement

2. Arch over ball.
3. Bend or extend your legs in front.
4. Open your arms to the side as if making the letter "T." Your head is supported by the ball.
5. Relax for 10–15 breaths.

Balancing Ball Tips

◆ If you have a back injury, please leave this stretch out.

◆ If you're not accustomed to arching, you may experience some dizziness especially when you come out of the stretch. Please rise slowly.

The Least You Need to Know

◆ These restorative stretches slow you down so you can sit quietly to explore imbalances in your body and your life.

◆ In some cases, muscle imbalance can alter your alignment, setting off the downward spiral that leads to injuries.

◆ The fitness ball makes the perfect prop for stretching because it lifts you off the floor.

◆ Stretching on the ball is especially beneficial if you have limited range of motion—have trouble getting on and off the floor.

◆ You can take the ball to work with you.

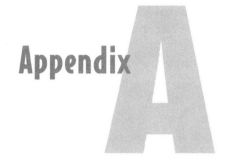

Appendix A

Glossary

This appendix contains words or common anatomy terms used in this book to enhance your ball training—or training in your local gym. Learn them and you're on your way to getting your best ball body.

abductors   Muscles of the outer thighs that move the legs away from the body and co-contract with adductors to assist in balance.

adductors   Muscles of the inner thigh that move the legs toward the midline of the body; they co-contract with abductors to assist in balance.

anti-burst balls   Rather than bursting, when a burst-resistance ball is punctured, the ball deflates slowly, preventing injury.

balance   The foundation for all movements. Specifically, balance and muscle contraction are an integral part of physical movement. Balance also requires a collaborative effort among the inner ear, eyes, muscles, and the brain to coordinate the body's position in space.

biceps brachii   Muscles of the upper front arm.

body composition   A method measuring fat to lean muscle in your body.

burst-balls   If a sharp object punctures a burst-ball, it deflates quickly, dropping the user to the floor.

cardiorespiratory fitness (or steady-rate endurance)   Fitness for the heart, lungs, and blood vessels. To get heart-pumping benefits, engage in aerobic exercise for 20–60 minutes in a continuous time frame or an intermittent minimum of 10-minute bouts accumulated throughout the day at least three times a week.

degenerated disc   A chronic weakening and thinning of a disc to the point that it can no longer provide a shock-absorbing cushion between vertebrae. As a result, the spinal bones may suffer bone spurs and terribly painful misalignment.

deltoids   The shoulder muscles that are arranged in layers: The anterior deltoid wraps in front, the medial deltoid wraps over the mid-shoulder, and the posterior deltoid wraps from the back.

fitness   Defined by the American Council of Sports Medicine as four elements: cardiorespiratory, strength, flexibility, and body composition.

fitness ball (also known as the stability ball, Swiss ball, and Resist-a-ball)   A large, heavy duty, inflatable ball on which strength exercises and stretches can be performed.

flexibility   A fitness element acquired through stretching. ACSM recommends stretching all major muscle groups at least two to three days a week. Stretching falls under two categories: static and dynamic. Static stretching holds a stretch for a certain period of time such as yoga; whereas, dynamic stretching moves your body through a stretch, such as Pilates.

functional fitness   A type of fitness that builds strength in movement, training your body so it is spatially aware of its position at any given moment.

gluteus maximus   The outermost of the three gluteal muscles and the biggest muscle of your buttocks.

hamstrings   The three muscles making up the back thighs: biceps femoris, semitendinosus, and semimembranosus.

herniated disc   A chronic weakening of the outer sheath of a spinal disc. As a result, the gel-like contents of the disc bulges, pressing on a nerve exiting the spine and causing mild to severe pain.

hip-pelvis complex   This is a group of numerous muscles and bones that connect the legs to the pelvis. This area directly influences the spine's position, so it's vitally important that exercises or stretches be performed with the pelvis in a stable (neutral) position. When training with a stable pelvis, the abdominals are strengthened, which supports the lower back, helping to relieve its workload.

latissimus dorsi   A broad back muscle that wraps from the back to the front ribs to provide trunk support in certain movements.

multifidus   A posterior stabilizing spine muscle, spanning three layers deep and runs the length of your spine, from the sacrum to the cervical vertebrae.

neutral spine   Proper spine alignment. If your spine is properly aligned, so, too, are your ligaments, tendons, muscles, and discs, enabling all systems to operate at peak performance because the whole body is under the least amount of stress, lessening the chances of injury.

pelvic floor muscles   These muscles assist in stabilizing your spine. The pelvic floors span five layers deep to cross through the bottom of the pelvis, from the pubic bone to the coccyx (anus) —imagine a hammock—and from butt bone to butt bone (you sit on these bones).

Pilates method   This is a smarter strategy to amazing abs, long and lean legs, and a lengthened body with perfect posture. Pilates, pronounced "puh-LAH-teez," is a total mind and body workout invented by Joseph Pilates (1880–1967).

Pilates breath   Inhaling through the nose to open up the rib cage, laterally, without the belly rising and exhaling deeply through the mouth to purge every last breath from the lungs. This lengthened exhalation is used to trigger the deep abdominal, the transverse, along with the other stabilizing muscles of the spine.

Pilates exercises   About 500 exercises which include —34 in a mat class. Exercises can be performed on a variety of machines with an instructor: the Universal Reformer, the Cadillac, the Wunda Chair, the Low and High Barrels, the Wall, the Mat, Ped-a-Pul, and the Magic Circle.

Pilates, Joseph (1880–1967) German-born body healer who based his method on both Eastern and Western philosophies, everything from yoga to Grecian sports.

postural training Training that includes strengthening the middle muscles to enhance posture, protecting the spine, and heightening body awareness as the mind and body unconsciously work to stabilize the body's center of gravity—both on the ball and in life.

posture Body alignment. Proper posture means aligning the body so that it can perform an action with maximum efficiency and minimum wear.

powerhouse A word coined by Joseph Pilates and used to describe the area of muscles that is the body's center. It forms a continuous band of muscles wrapping around the waist, from the bottom of the rib cage to the hip bones, and is comprised of the abdominals, back, and hips.

prone A body position that trains the body in a face down position and is ideal for strengthening the muscles of the backside.

proprioception A sense of where the body is in its space. Ball training strengthens proprioception and enhances the brain to body connection.

quadriceps The four muscles of the front of the thigh, originating on the thigh bone or femur and running in various directions past the knee: The rectus femoris is the big muscle of the front thigh; vastus medialis attaches to the inner front portion of the femur; the vastus lateralis attaches to the outer front; and the vastus intermedius attaches between the two.

scapulae Shoulder blades. A pair of winged-bones that float on the upper spine, directly influencing the position of the shoulders and part of a complex of bones and muscles that attach the arms to the spine.

scoliosis A condition of the spine, causing lateral displacement in the lower and upper parts of the back; it forms an "S"-like curve in the back. Some people are born with it while others engage in one-sided activities that can alter the spinal curves.

six guiding principles The foundation of Pilates, which can be applied to everyday life: centering, control, concentration, flow, precision, and breathing.

spine Anatomical life support. The column of spinal bones or vertebrae that enable movement. The home of the life force—the spinal cord.

stabilizing spinal muscles The transverse, multifidus, and pelvic floors, which act like a brace for your spine, providing spinal stabilization.

strength The foundation for muscular fitness. It includes the ability to lift a heavy object and the ability to repeatedly use a muscle—muscular endurance. (A balanced fitness formula requires both.)

supine A face up position.

transversus abdominis (or transverse) The deepest of all abdominal muscles, which sits deep in the trunk. Because of its anatomical wrap around the spine, the transverse stabilizes the spine as it contracts, forming a deep girdle of spinal support by pulling the abdominal wall near your spine.

triceps brachii The muscles of the upper-back arm.

Quick Workouts: Multi-Muscle Training

Sometimes you just don't have time to train every major muscle in your body. That's where this quick workout comes in. This collection of exercises targets every major muscle in your body, so you can walk away feeling complete; it's the quickest way to overall body slimming results. Try to sweat it out with some form of cardio for at least 30 minutes, five to six times a week if you want to see serious fat reduction results. After that, do the following multi-muscle exercises—I promise 10 minutes tops!

The following can be modified or intensified to meet your fitness level.

Ball wall squat (pages 62-63)

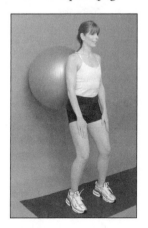
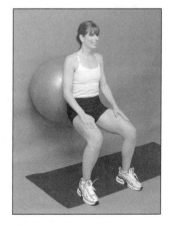

Ball single leg lunge (page 73)

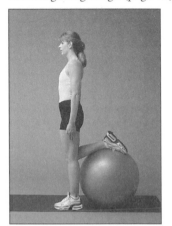 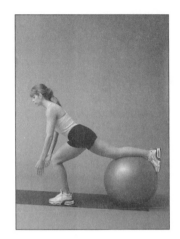

Stationary ball plank (page 75)

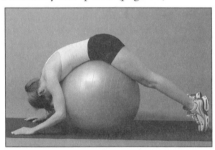 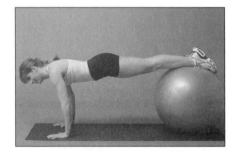

Stationary ball push-up (page 78)

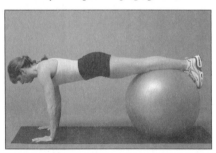 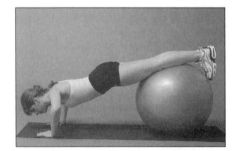

Spinal ball extension (page 79)

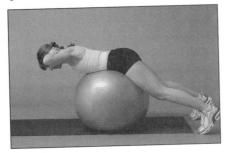
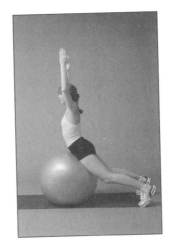

Drape (page 41)

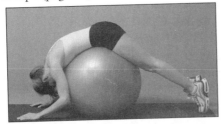

Ball bridge with leg curls and leg extensions (pages 81-82)

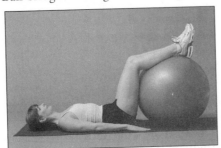
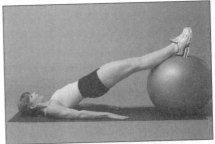

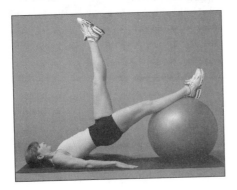
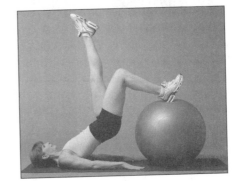

Lower back stretch (page 149)

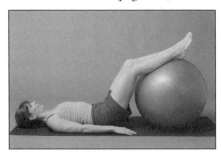 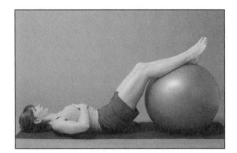

Quick Workouts: Just Abs!

Just because you're crunched for time, doesn't mean you have to blow off your much-needed abdominal work. The following are five abdominal ball exercises that will transform any old pooch. This exercises target all of your abdominal muscles mainly because variety is the spice of life and key to making your ab routine more effective. Again, add some cardio for at least 30 minutes, five to six days a week, and then do the following abdominal ball exercises.

The following can be modified or intensified to meet your fitness level.

Abdominal ball curl (page 38)

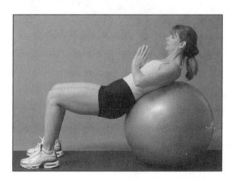 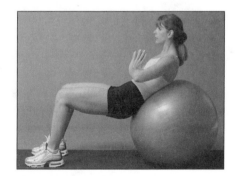

Abdominal ball oblique curl (page 60)

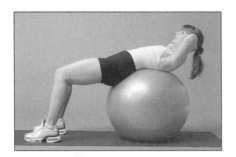 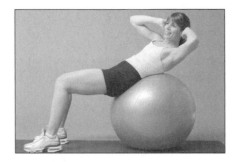

Inner thigh squeeze with abdominal curl (page 83)

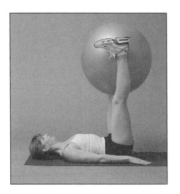 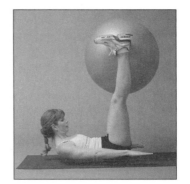

Reverse ball curl (page 84)

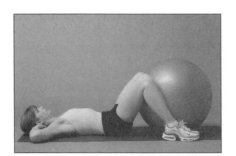 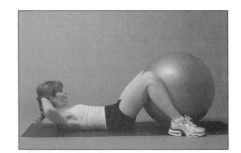

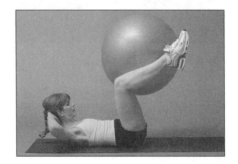

Scissor ball rotation (page 85)

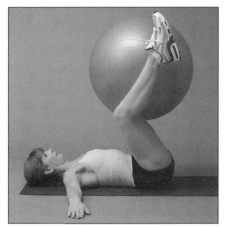 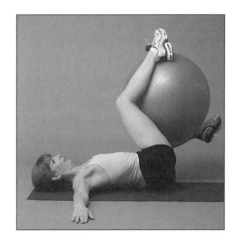

Beat Belly Fat with the Ball

It's belly time. To get awesome results on the ball you need a extra oomph in your workout. So below is a collection of six exercises for serious ab results. This workout adds some mutli-muscle moves yet specifically targets your core: abdominal and back muscles.

Abdominal ball curl (page 59)

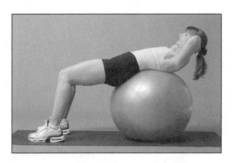 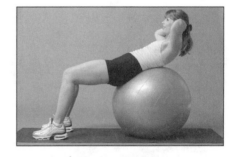

Abdominal ball oblique curl (page 60)

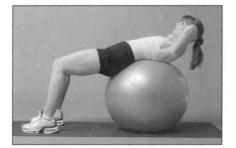 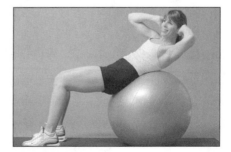

Spinal ball extension (page 40)

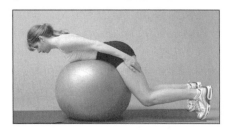 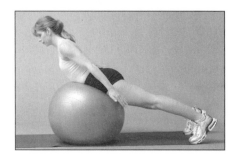

Drape over the ball (page 41)

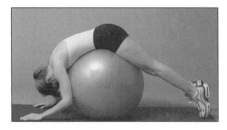

Spinal ball extension with legs lift (page 57)

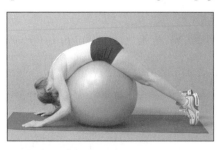 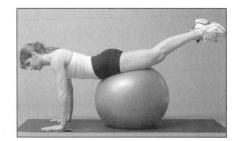

Ball bridge on floor (page 44)

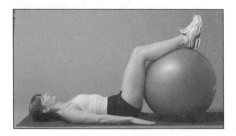 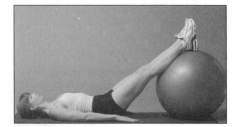

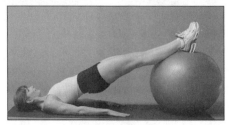

Ball bridge with leg curls and leg extensions (pages 81-82)

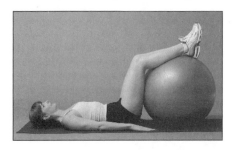
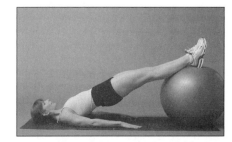

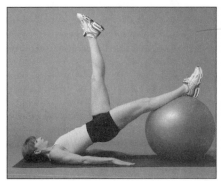
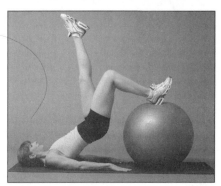

Reverse ball curl (page 84)

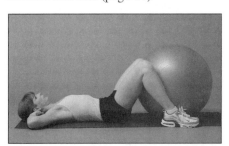
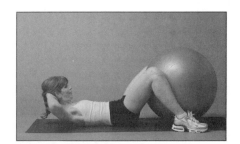

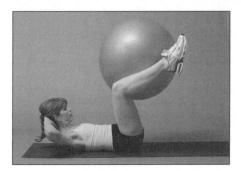

Appendix E

Myths and Mysteries About Abdominal Training

Picturing the anatomy of your abs is fairly simple concept if you just imagine an onion peel—layers and layers provide the onion its shape and strength just like the layers and layers of muscle that make up your torso. The deepest abdominal muscle is the transverse abdominis, which run horizontally around your middle and stabilizes your spine; it contacts or pulls inward with the help of other abdominal muscles, which are layered on top. For example, the internal obliques run diagonally from your pelvis to the lower ribs and rest on top of the transverse while your external obliques run from the ribs to your pelvis and sit on top of the internal obliques. The most superficial ab muscle, the rectus abdominis, runs from the top of your pubic bone to your sternum.

1. **Myth:** Crunches will get rid of flabby abs?

   The lowdown: While crunches can be part of an anti ab flab campaign, this exercise alone can not get rid of the flab. Spot training or reducing fat to one area of the body is never an effective way to lose overall inches. You need to do a total body strength workout (the ones, for example, in Chapters 4 through 5) to increase overall lean muscle mass and reduce fat. Most important, you need to focus on strengthening your core as a unit, meaning engaging all of your abdominal muscles. Plus, you need to add a consistent cardio routine to your week at least 5 to 6 days a week of 30 minutes to 60 minutes if you want to see visible fat reducing results.

2. **Myth:** To streamline your abdominals, you need to do ab exercises everyday?

   The lowdown: Your abdominal muscles are endurance muscles and have the ability to recover fairly quickly; however, they are a muscle and need time to recuperate just like any other muscle in your body. Therefore, you should train your abs every other day; letting them rest in between workouts.

3. **Myth:** You should do at least a hundred crunches to get six-pack abs.

   The lowdown: Again, because your abdominals are endurance muscles and have greater endurance than most muscle groups, that doesn't translate to "no pain-no gain" theory! If you're doing abs correctly, meaning that you're focusing on your spinal form and using slow and controlled movements, you should feel your abs working. There should be no reason to do more than three sets of 12-25 reps. Remember, quality over quantity!

4. **Myth:** You should train your abs at the end of your workout?

   The lowdown: Rather than focus on just your abdominals, think multi-muscle workouts! In each multi-muscle workout, you will engage in a variety of exercises that also activate your core. Not only will you burn more calories, but you'll save time as well. But if you need a quick ab workout, then, yes, you can do your abs at the end of each workout. However, it's perfectly okay to get your ab work in early, if you have a tendency to roll up your mat early.

Index

A

abdominals
  balls
    curls, 38, 59
    oblique curl exercises, 60
  fitness benefits, 14
  inner thigh ball squeeze with abdominal
    curl exercise, 83
  obliques
    curl exercise, 60
    muscles, 33
  Pilates, 102
  reverse ball curl exercise, 84
abductors, 70, 93
ACE (American Council of Exercise), 6
ACSM (American College of Sports
  Medicine), 12
adductors stretch exercise, 70, 93, 149
advanced exercises, 69-70
  ball bridge with leg curls and leg extensions,
    81-82
  ball plié wall squat with upright row, 70-72,
    93
  ball single leg lunge, 73

ball wall squat with biceps curl, 71
inner thigh ball squeeze with abdominal
  curl, 83
one arm standing row with single leg ball
  squat, 74
reverse ball curl, 84
scissor ball rotation, 85
spinal ball extension, 79-80
stationary ball
  pike, 77
  plank, 75-76
  push-up, 78
aerobic exercises, 12
American College of Sports Medicine (ACSM),
  12
American Council of Exercise (ACE), 6
anti-burst balls, 9
arms
  ball wall squat with biceps curl exercise, 71
  one arm standing row
    with ball exercise, 58
    with single leg ball squat exercise, 74
  seated ball
    bent-over fly exercise, 53
    bicep curl exercise, 49

front raise exercise, 51
lateral raise exercise, 52
postural exercise, 34-36
triceps extension exercise, 50
spinal ball, extension exercise, 56, 80
supine ball bridge
    with chest press exercise, 54
    with fly exercise, 55

B

backs
    ball plié wall squat with upright row
        exercise, 70-72, 93
    injuries, 112
    muscles, 41
    neutral position, 20-21
    pains
        exercises, 125-136
        fighting aches, 124
        lifestyle effects, 123
        lumbar, 123
        reconditioning, 122
        self-diagnosis, 124-125
        therapy choices, 121-122
        therapy guidelines, 137
    pelvis, 21-22
    shoulder blades, 22-23
    spine basics, 20
balance
    fitness ball, 6, 14
    single leg standing, 73
balanced bodies, 11-12
    building with fitness ball, 13-14
        balance, 14
        body sense training, 15
        posture, 14-15

cardiorespiratory fitness, 12
    flexibility, 13
    life style effects, 16
    strength, 12-13
ball beats exercise, Pilates, 115-116
ball bridge
    on floor exercises, 44
    with leg curl exercises, 66
    with leg curls and leg extensions exercises,
        81-82
ball curls, abdominals, 38
ball plié wall squat
    exercises, 64
    with upright row exercises, 70-72, 93
ball rocking, seated ball postural exercises,
    32-33
ball sideline outer thigh work exercises, 65
ball single leg lunge exercises, 73
ball wall squat
    exercises, 62-63
    with biceps curl exercises, 71
beginner exercises, 29-30
    abdominal ball curls, 38
    ball bridge on floor, 44
    cross ball extension, 42
    drape over ball, 41
    Pilates, 97-98
    seated ball postural
        ball rocking, 32-33
        finding neutral spine, 30-31
        leg and arm raises, 34-36
    stationary ball plank, 43
    supine ball
        bridge, 39
        extension, 40
    walking down ball, 36-37
bent-over flys, seated ball exercise, 53

biceps
  ball wall squat with biceps curl exercise, 71
  seated ball curl exercise, 49
bodies
  composition, measuring body fat, 13
  sense, fitness ball training, 15
breathing, 30, 93
burst-resistant balls, 9
buttocks
  ball bridge with leg curls and leg extensions exercise, 81-82
  ball plié wall squat with upright row exercise, 70-72, 93
  ball single leg lunge exercise, 73
  Pilates
    ball beats exercise, 115-116
    kick front and back exercise, 113
    leg ball circles exercise, 114

C

cardio exercises, 12
cardiorespiratory fitness, 12
CDC (Center for Disease Control), 12
Center for Disease Control (CDC), 12
center of gravity, 15
centering, Pilates, 92
cervical curves, 20
chest
  stationary ball push-up exercise, 78
  supine ball bridge press exercise, 54
cleaning fitness balls, 8
coccygeal vertebraes, 21
Complete Idiot's Guide to Pilates, The, 100
concentration, Pilates, 92
control, Pilates, 92
cross ball extensions, 42

curls
  abdominal ball
    exercise, 59
    oblique exercise, 60
  ball bridge with leg exercise, 66
  inner thigh ball squeeze with abdominal curl exercise, 83
  reverse ball curl exercise, 84
  seated ball bicep exercise, 49

D-E

degenerated discs, 124
double-leg stretch exercise, Pilates, 109
drape over ball exercises, 41

endurance, steady-rate, 12
erector spinae, 24, 41
exercise balls. *See* fitness balls
exercises
  advanced, 69-70
    ball bridge with leg curls and leg extensions, 81-82
    ball plié wall squat with upright row, 70-72, 93
    ball single leg lunge, 73
    ball wall squat with biceps curl, 71
    inner thigh ball squeeze with abdominal curl, 83
    one arm standing row with single leg ball squat, 74
    reverse ball curl, 84
    scissor ball rotation, 85
    spinal ball extension, 79
    spinal ball extension with triceps kickback, 80
    stationary ball pike, 77
    stationary ball plank, 43, 75-76
    stationary ball push-up, 78

back pain, 125
   hamstring stretch, 128
   lower back stretch, 126
   moving legs with stable spine, 127
   pectoral and latissimus stretch, 129
   plank, 135
   raise ball overhead, 136
   seated hip flexion to seated knee extension, 132
   seated pelvic tilts, 131
   seated spine stretch, 130
   small rotation with neutral spine, 133-134
beginner, 29-30
   abdominal ball curls, 38
   ball bridge on floor, 44
   cross ball extension, 42
   drape over ball, 41
   Pilates, 97-98
   seated ball postural, 30-36
   stationary ball plank, 43
   supine ball bridge, 39
   supine ball extension, 40
   walking down ball, 36-37
intermediate, 47-48
   abdominal ball curl, 59
   abdominal ball oblique curl, 60
   ball bridge with leg curl, 66
   ball plié wall squat, 64
   ball sideline outer thigh work, 65
   ball wall squat, 62-63
   one arm standing row with ball, 58
   seated ball bent-over fly, 53
   seated ball bicep curl, 49
   seated ball front raise, 51
   seated ball lateral raise, 52
   seated ball tricep extension, 50
   spinal ball extension, 56
   spinal ball extension with leg lift, 57

stationary ball plank, 61
supine ball bridge with chest press, 54
supine ball bridge with fly, 55
Pilates
   double-leg stretch, 109
   fab five, 98
   fitness ball, 95
   hundred on the ball, 99-100
   lateral breathing, 94
   leg circles, 103-104
   rolling like ball, 105-106
   rollup, 101-102
   Saw, 111-112
   Seal, 117
   side kick ball series, 113-116
   single-leg stretch, 107-108
   spine stretch, 110
   "V" stance, 98
restorative ball
   adductor stretch, 149
   gluteal stretch, 150
   hamstring stretch, 147
   lower back stretch, 149
   pectoral stretch, 143
   prone quadriceps stretch, 152
   seated back stretch, 142
   seated buttocks and hamstrings stretch, 154
   seated chest stretch, 142-143
   seated lateral trunk stretch, 145
   seated neck stretch, 141, 156
   seated rotation stretch, 144
   sideline stretch, 151
   spinal twist, 148
   standing back stretch, 155
   standing shoulder stretch at wall, 155
   supine arm circles, 146
   supine spinal traction, 153, 156
   thread the needle stretch, 150

F

fat, measuring body fat, 13
feet positioning, 53
fitness
    balanced body, 12
        building with fitness ball, 13-15
        cardiorespiratory, 12
        flexibility, 13
        strength, 12-13
    functional, 5-7
    life style effects, 16
    measuring body fat, 13
fitness balls
    balanced body fitness, 13-14
        balance, 14
        body sense training, 15
        posture, 14-15
    cleaning, 8
    functional fitness, 5-7
    overcoming plateau states, 7-8
    Pilates, 95
    pitfalls, 25
    posture guidelines, 24-25
    precautions, 8-9
    selection, 8-11
flat back postures, pelvis, 22
flexibility, balanced body fitness, 13
flow, Pilates, 92
flys
    seated ball exercise, 53
    supine ball bridge with fly exercise, 55
front raises, seated ball exercise, 51
functional fitness, 5-7

G–H

gluteal stretch exercise, restorative ball, 150
good posture, 20

hamstring stretch exercise
    back pains, 128
    restorative ball, 147
healing processes, muscle stretching, 139-140
health, exercise benefit studies, 12
herniated discs, 124
hundred on the ball, Pilates, 99-100

I

inflation fitness ball, 8
inner thigh ball squeeze with abdominal curl
    exercises, 83
Institute of Medicine (IOM), 12
intermediate exercises, 47-48
    abdominal ball
        curl, 59
        oblique curl, 60
    ball bridge with leg curl, 66
    ball plié wall squat, 64
    ball sideline outer thigh work, 65
    ball wall squat, 62-63
    one arm standing row with ball, 58
    seated ball
        bent-over fly, 53
        bicep curl, 49
        front raise, 51
        lateral raise, 52
        triceps extension, 50
    spinal ball extension, 56-57
    stationary ball plank, 61

supine ball bridge
with chest press, 54
with fly, 55
IOM (Institute of Medicine), 12

J-K

joints, multitasking exercises, 79
Journal of Medicine and Science in Sports and Exercise, 14

Katzmarzyk, Ph.D., Peter T., abdominal fitness benefits, 14
kick front and back exercise, Pilates, 113
KleinVogelbach, Dr. Susan, Swiss ball, 6

L

lat muscles, 24
lateral breathing, 93-94
lateral raises, seated ball exercise, 52
latissimus dorsi muscles, 24
lats, one arm standing row with single leg ball squat exercise, 74
legs
ball bridge with leg curls
exercise, 66
leg extensions exercise, 81-82
ball circles exercise, Pilates, 114
ball plié wall squat with upright row exercise, 70-72, 93
ball sideline outer thigh work exercise, 65
ball single leg lunge exercise, 73
ball wall squat with biceps curl exercise, 71
inner thigh ball squeeze with abdominal curl exercise, 83
one arm standing row with single leg ball squat exercise, 74

Pilates
ball beats exercise, 115-116
double-leg stretch, 109
kick front and back exercise, 113
leg ball circles exercise, 114
leg circles, 103-104
single-leg stretch, 107-108
quadriceps, 62
reverse ball curl exercise, 84
scissor ball rotation exercise, 85
seated ball postural exercise, 34-36
single leg standing, 73
spinal ball extension lift exercise, 57
stationary ball plank with leg extension, 76
life style
effects on back, 123
effects on health, 16
lower back
pains, 123
stretch
back pains, 126
exercise, restorative ball, 126, 149
lumbar
back pains, 123
exercises, 125-136
fighting aches, 124
lifestyle effects, 123
self-diagnosis, 124-125
spines, 20
lunges, ball single leg exercise, 73

M

mat exercises, Pilates, 91
mid-deltoid muscles, ball plié wall squat with upright row exercise, 70-72, 93

middle muscles
 fitness ball guidelines, 24-25
 posture, 23-24
moving legs with stable spine exercise, back pains, 127
multi-muscle training, 69-70
 ball bridge with leg curls and leg extensions exercise, 81-82
 ball plié wall squat with upright row, 70-72, 93
 ball single leg lunge, 73
 ball wall squat with biceps curl, 71
 inner thigh ball squeeze with abdominal curl exercise, 83
 one arm standing row with single leg ball squat, 74
 reverse ball curl exercise, 84
 scissor ball rotation exercise, 85
 spinal ball extension, 79-80
 stationary ball
  pike, 77
  plank, 75-76
  push-up, 78
multifidus muscles, 23
muscles
 back, 41
 posture, 23-25
 stress
  restorative ball, 140-156
  stretching, 139-140

N-O

National Institute of Health, 12
neutral spine positions, 20-21, 30-31

obliques, abdominal curl exercise, 60
one arm standing row
 with ball exercises, 58
 with single leg ball squat exercises, 74

P

pectorals
 latissimus stretch exercise, back pains, 129
 stretch exercise, restorative ball, 143
pelvis
 floor muscles, 23
 pelvic tilts, back pain, 126, 131
 spine influence, 21-22
Pilates
 beginnings, 90
 definition, 89-90
 exercises
  double-leg stretch, 109
  hundred on the ball, 99-100
  leg circles, 103-104
  rolling like ball, 105-106
  rollup, 101-102
  Saw, 111-112
  Seal, 117
  side kick ball series, 113-116
  single-leg stretch, 107-108
  spine stretch, 110
 fab five exercises, 98
 fitness ball, 95-98
 lateral breathing exercises, 94
 principles, 91-93
 strengthing, 90-91
 stretching, 90-91
 "V" stance, 98
Pilates, Joseph
 beginnings, 90
 method, 89

plank exercises
    back pains, 135
    hand position, 43
    stationary ball, 43
        pike, 77
        plank, 61, 75-76
        push-up, 78
plateau states, 7-8
posture
    fitness ball
        body fitness, 14-15
        guidelines, 24-25
    harmony, Pilates, 90-91
    improving, 19-20
    muscles, 23-24
    seated ball postural exercise, finding neutral
        spine, 30-31
    spine, 20
        neutral position, 20-21
        pelvis, 21-22
        shoulder blades, 22-23
powerhouse, Pilates, 92
precautions, 8-9
precision, Pilates, 92
principles, Pilates, 91-93
prone positions, 40
prone quadriceps stretch exercise, restorative
    ball, 152
proprioception, 15
pumps, inflating fitness ball, 8
push-ups, stationary ball exercise, 78

Q-R

quadriceps, 62
quads, 62

raise ball overhead exercises, back pains, 136
reconditioning, back, 122
rectus femoris, 62
Resist-a-balls. *See* fitness balls
restorative ball, 140
    adductor stretch, 149
    gluteal stretch, 150
    hamstring stretch, 147
    lower back stretch, 149
    pectoral stretch, 143
    prone quadriceps stretch, 152
    seated back stretch, 142
    seated buttocks and hamstrings stretch, 154
    seated chest stretch, 142-143
    seated lateral trunk stretch, 145
    seated neck stretch, 141, 156
    seated rotation stretch, 144
    sideline stretch, 151
    spinal twist, 148
    standing back stretch, 155
    standing shoulder stretch at wall, 155
    supine arm circles, 146
    supine spinal traction, 153, 156
    thread the needle stretch, 150
reverse ball curl exercises, 84
rhomboid muscles, 24
rolling like ball exercise, Pilates, 105-106
rollups, Pilates, 101-102

S

sacral vertebraes, 21
sacrums, 21
Sanzo, Karen, 122
saw exercise, Pilates, 111-112
scapulae, 22-23
scissor ball rotation exercises, 85

scoliosis, 124

Seal exercises, Pilates, 117

seated back stretch exercise, restorative ball, 142

seated ball
bent-over fly exercises, 53
biceps curl exercises, 49
biceps triceps extension exercises, 50
front raise exercises, 51
lateral raise exercises, 52
postural exercises
ball rocking, 32-33
finding neutral spine, 30-31
leg and arm raises, 34-36

seated buttocks and hamstrings stretch exercise, restorative ball, 154

seated chest stretch exercise, restorative ball, 142-143

seated hip flexion to seated knee extension exercise, back pains, 132

seated lateral trunk stretch exercise, restorative ball, 145

seated neck stretch exercise, restorative ball, 141, 156

seated pelvic tilts exercise, back pains, 131

seated rotation stretch exercise, restorative ball, 144

seated spine stretch exercise, back pains, 130

serratus anterior muscles, 24

severe arch positions, pelvis, 22

shoulders, 22-23, 78

side kick ball series, Pilates
ball beats, 115-116
kick front and back, 113
leg ball circles, 114

sideline stretch exercise, restorative ball, 151

single-leg stretch exercise, Pilates, 107-108

small rotation with neutral spine exercise, back pains, 133-134

spine, 20
ball extension
exercises, 56, 79
with leg lift exercises, 57
with triceps kickback exercises, 80
fitness ball guidelines, 24-25
neutral position, 20-21
pains
exercises, 125-136
fighting aches, 124
lifestyle effects, 123
lumbar, 123
reconditioning, 122
self-diagnosis, 124-125
therapy choices, 121-122
therapy guidelines, 137
pelvis, 21-22
Pilates
ball beats exercise, 115-116
seal exercise, 117
spine stretch, 110
seated ball postural exercise, 30-31
shoulder blades, 22-23
spinal ball extension, 56
exercise, 79
with triceps kickback exercise, 80
stretch exercise, Pilates, 110
twist exercise, restorative ball, 148

squats
ball plié wall
exercise, 64
squat with upright row exercise, 70-72, 93
ball wall
exercise, 62-63
squat with biceps curl exercise, 71
one arm standing row with single leg ball squat exercise, 74

stability balls. *See* fitness balls

standing back stretch exercise, restorative ball, 155

standing shoulder stretch at wall exercise, restorative ball, 155

stationary ball
  pike exercises, 77
  plank exercises, 43, 61, 75-76
  push-up exercises, 78

steady-rate endurance, 12

strength
  balanced body fitness, 12-13
  Pilates, 90-91

stress
  restorative ball, 140
    adductor stretch, 149
    gluteal stretch, 150
    hamstring stretch, 147
    lower back stretch, 149
    pectoral stretch, 143
    prone quadriceps stretch, 152
    seated back stretch, 142
    seated buttocks and hamstrings stretch, 154
    seated chest stretch, 142-143
    seated lateral trunk stretch, 145
    seated neck stretch, 141, 156
    seated rotation stretch, 144
    sideline stretch, 151
    spinal twist, 148
    standing back stretch, 155
    standing shoulder stretch at wall, 155
    supine arm circles, 146
    supine spinal traction, 153, 156
    thread the needle stretch, 150

stretching muscles
  Pilates, 90-91
  restorative ball, 140-156
  stress reliever, 139-140

studies, weight loss, 12

supine arm circles exercise, restorative ball, 146

supine ball bridge, 39
  with chest press exercises, 54
  with fly exercises, 55

supine ball extensions, 40

supine spinal traction exercise, restorative ball, 153, 156

Swiss balls, 6. *See also* fitness balls

synergistic movements, Pilates, 91

T

therapies, back, 121-122, 137

thighs
  ball plié wall squat with upright row exercise, 70-72, 93
  ball sideline outer thigh work, 65
  inner thigh ball squeeze with abdominal curl exercise, 83
  reverse ball curl exercise, 84
  scissor ball rotation exercise, 85

thoracic curves, 20

thread the needle stretch exercise, restorative ball, 150

transverse muscles, 23

transversus abdominis, 23

trap muscles, 24

trapezius muscles, 24

triceps
  seated ball extension exercise, 50
  spinal ball extension with triceps kickback exercise, 80

trunk muscles, 23-25

U-V

U.S. Surgeon General, 12

"V" stance, Pilates, 98
vastus intermedius, 62
vastus lateralis, 62
vastus medialis, 62
vertebraes
    coccygeal, 21
    lumbar, 20
    sacral, 21

W-X-Y-Z

waist, scissor ball rotation exercise, 85
walking down ball, 36-37
weight loss, aerobic exercise studies, 12

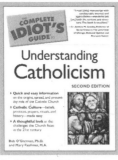
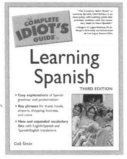
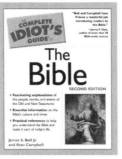
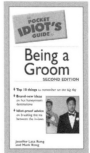
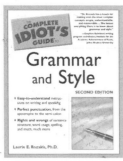
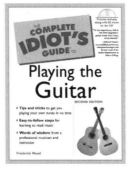
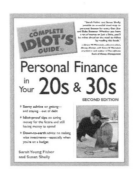
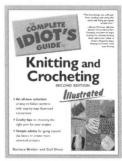
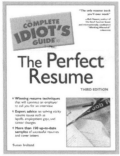
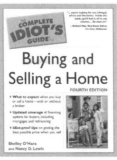
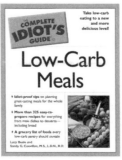
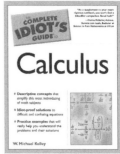